The Exceptional Nurse

Tales from the Trenches of Truly Resilient
Nurses Working with Disabilities

Edited by

Donna Carol Maheady, EdD, ARNP

D1371988

Stories of courageous nurses who have pursued their profession despite conditions that others might consider impossible obstacles are presented in this book. Their special insights into the needs of others make them truly exceptional nurses. I applaud Dr. Maheady for bringing these stories together to inspire nurses and those who would seek a career in nursing.

Karen Kelly, EdD, RN, NEA-BC, Director, Continuing Education & Associate Professor, School of Nursing, Southern Illinois University Edwardsville, Edwardsville, IL

This book offers inspiration and resources for when times get tough. And, shown me that I am not alone! Nurses share their hearts and how to make it through darkness into the light. Whether your challenge is yet to come, or is here, this is a book of guidance and encouragement. I've had epilepsy most of my life and learned to accept my challenge and use it as a tool to bless others—colleagues, patients, and families; who have shared stories about having seizures. It is possible to live a normal life with epilepsy and be a nurse."

Erica Laney, RN, Community Hospice of Northeast Florida, Jacksonville, Florida

A disability may be in my future. I wonder how my college would treat me. When nursing faculty and students have disabilities, the university demonstrates a commitment to diversity and equal opportunity. We would hope that a caring program cares for its own. Our first question should be "how can we help you realize your goal?"

Jill E. Winland-Brown, EdD, FNP-BC, DPNAP, Professor and Family Nurse Practitioner, Christine E. Lynn College of Nursing, Florida Atlantic University, ANA Ethics and Human Rights Advisory Board

A career in nursing is a calling. Nursing school is a challenge. Nursing school with a disability is surmountable if the nursing student and school faculty work together to meet the challenge. This book illustrates how that challenge can and has been met. As a nurse with spina bifida who uses a wheelchair, I know it can be done.

Marianne Haugh RN, MSN, CRRN, Staff Educator at Shriners Hospitals for Children-Chicago, Clinical Supervisor for William Rainey Harper College and the University of St. Francis-Joliet

The stories are so compelling. These nurses have not just survived but thrived to overcome the difficulties faced by life-long or unforeseen disabilities.... beyond impressive journeys. It is important to understand that if you are discriminated against there is a process that takes TIME. There is no protection for discrimination and harassment. How do we protect someone when an investigation is underway? The book's suggestion to plan yearly check-ups---consider the 'what ifs', plan for the unknown future and not take any day for granted will certainly help.

Paula McWilliam, Ed.D, NNP, Associate Nursing Professor, St. Joseph's College. Affiliate Nursing Research Professor, University of New Hampshire, Advocate/mentor for nurses and nursing students with disabilities www.ExceptionalNurse.com

DEDICATION

To my daughter, Lauren, thank you for teaching me so much.
I love you big

To my husband, Tom Gili, my love and thanks
for your ongoing support of my work.

To nursing professors, nurses and administrators who have supported a
nursing student or nurse with a disability, I am thankful.

And to all of the nurses with disabilities
who had the courage to share their stories, I am thankful.
Your stories will help so many other nurses and nursing students.

May more nurses and nursing students with disabilities find
a safe place to land and an opportunity work.

"May the road rise up to meet you
May the wind be always at your back
May the sun shine warm upon your face
And the rain fall soft upon your fields
And until we meet again
May God hold you in the palm of his hand"
(Irish Blessing)

CONTENTS

INTRODUCTION

By Donna Carol Maheady, ARNP, EdD

During a recent interview, I was asked if the tide is turning in favor of nurses with disabilities. Before responding, I reflected over the many years since I created www.ExceptionalNurse.com and then said, "I wouldn't say that the tide has turned yet. I would describe conditions as a meandering river or stream. In some areas, the gains have been substantial. In other areas, there is barely a ripple." Regardless of remarkable experience and skills, nurses with disabilities can feel diminished at work.

Exact numbers of nurses with disabilities are not available for many reasons. Some nurses do not disclose their disability due to fear of job termination—often scared silent. Others are involved in lawsuits and are advised not to share information.

The National Nurses Survey in 2008 reported that 14,102 nurses listed disability or illness as a reason for employer or position change (U.S. Department of Health & Human Services, 2008). Anecdotal reports show that nurses have disabilities that mirror the general population. Additionally, nurses report being injured by lifting patients, through violence inflicted by patients or exposure to latex, hepatitis and HIV.

The Americans with Disabilities Act was passed in 1990 and amended in 2008 in an effort to level the playing field for people with disabilities. The law and the meaning of reasonable accommodations have been interpreted differently over the years, resulting in inconsistencies in admission, hiring and retention decisions. A major change that Congress enacted when passing the Americans with Disabilities Act Amendments Act (ADAAA) is that nursing students may be protected based on actual or perceived impairments, whether or not their disabilities limit a major life activity (Dupler, et al, 2012).

In all my years of working as an advocate for nurses with disabilities, I have never heard of a nurse who *plans* to become disabled. Resources for parents of children with disabilities abound as well as guides for adults to learn to cope with being or becoming disabled. *But*, where do nurses turn?

Many Questions Exist

Where do nurses find support? Where do they find answers to questions like, "Should I disclose?" What are their legal entitlements to reasonable accommodation? Where do they find stethoscopes for hearing loss; real-time captioning services; computer screen readers for vision loss? Can vocational rehabilitation services help? Where do vocational rehabilitation counselors find information about options for nurses returning to work following disability? Where do parents of children with disabilities turn to find answers to whether or not they should encourage their child's interest in nursing? Where do nurses, administrators, educators and counselors find examples of nurses with disabilities who have continued to work with or without accommodations?

In this book, readers will find answers to these questions and more. First person accounts are included from nurses with various disabilities. Their stories are followed by commentaries from a wide range of professionals. The focus of the book is on the *abilities* of these nurses, not their limitations. Their stories—some long and some short— show how nurses can turn a disability into an integral part of their nursing care. Disability can be a force of giving and empowering in spite of the odds stacked against nurses with disabilities.

State vocational rehabilitation programs may be helpful in offering support to nurses or students with disabilities interested in a nursing career. A chapter includes information about working with state vocational rehabilitation programs and a guide to requesting services is included in the Appendix.

The stories demonstrate how nurses with disabilities do their work with and without accommodations, often by reinventing themselves. If they can't get in the front door, they go around to the side door.

The information is important reading for nurses at any point in their careers. Career planning needs to include the possibility of disability. Readers will also gain insight into the experience of nursing colleagues who become disabled or those who are hired with a disability.

Nurses and students with disabilities are encouraged to become resilient: Each chapter of the book is followed by recommendations to build resilience. Students with disabilities will be inspired to consider nursing as a career. And employers and nurse managers will be motivated to be more open to considering reasonable accommodation requests from nurses.

Now, let's get to work.

Donna Carol Maheady, ARNP, EdD, the mother of an adult daughter with autism and related disabilities, is a board certified pediatric nurse practitioner and an associate graduate faculty member in the Christine E. Lynn College of Nursing at Florida Atlantic University. Dr. Maheady has conducted research on the experiences of nursing students with disabilities, published numerous articles and is the author of Nursing Students with Disabilities Change the Course *(winner of the American Journal of Nursing 2004 Book of the Year Award)* and Leave No Nurse Behind: Nurses working with disAbilities. *She is the founder of the nonprofit resource network www.ExceptionalNurse.com and can be reached at ExceptionalNurse@aol.com.*

References

Dupler, A., Allen, C., Maheady, D., Fleming, S., Allen, M. (2012). Leveling the playing field for nursing students with disabilities: Implications of the Amendments to the Americans with Disabilities Act. *Journal of Nursing Education,* 51 (3), 140-144.

Maheady, D. (2003). *Nursing Students with Disabilities Change the Course.* River Edge, NJ: Exceptional Parent Press.

Maheady, D. (2006). *Leave No Nurse Behind: Nurses Working with Disabilities.* Lincoln, NE: iUniverse, Inc.

Sowers, J., & Smith, M. (2002). Disability as difference. *Journal of Nursing Education, 41* (8), 331-332.

U.S. Department of Health and Human Services, Bureau of Health Professions (2008). *The Registered Nurse Population: Findings from the 2008 National Sample Survey of Registered Nurses (Table 39).* Retrieved on May 8, 2014 at http://bhpr.hrsa.gov/healthworkforce/rnsurveys/rnsurveyfinal.pdf

Wood, D., Marshall, E.S. (2010). Nurses with disabilities working in hospital settings: Attitudes, concerns, and experiences of nurse leaders. *Journal of Professional Nursing,* 26(3), 182-187.

1 RESILIENCY
By Pamela Delis, RN, BS, MSN

The term "resiliency" inspires thoughts of positive attitude, perseverance, the ability to draw on support in overcoming difficulties, and the capacity to bounce back after a negative event. Resiliency allows a person to cope through everyday challenges, and through life-altering events. It suggests an inner strength, a desire to keep moving forward despite the odds. Resiliency is what makes for successful healing and rehabilitation in healthcare. Similarly, healthcare professionals encourage their patients to be resilient and draw on inner strength and support systems in their fight to overcome and adapt to health challenges.

Nurses and other health professionals display resiliency every day as they negotiate the demands and stressors of the healthcare environment. In this book, you will read the stories presented by nurses and nursing students who have faced or are facing healthcare challenges, and who, in spite of or because of these challenges, have proven they have the perseverance and inner strength to overcome the odds.

Inspiration from Others

Through the sharing of stories, these nurses hope to encourage others who may be facing their own challenges. In the 2010 article in the Journal of Nursing Research titled, "Storytelling: An Approach that Can Help to Develop Resilience," the authors East, Jackson, O'Brien and Peters (2010, p. 22) assert that storytelling is a "method that can celebrate survival and contribute to the resilience of storyteller, listener and others who engage with the story in subsequent published accounts." Through the sharing of stories, both teller and listener can gain valuable insight into the strengths and supportive mechanisms utilized to achieve positive outcomes following a challenging event. East, et al. (2010) purport that readers can "develop their resilience by learning and reflecting on...stories" (p. 20). Through another's tale, people can envision their own strengths and coping mechanisms, and identify their own supportive systems thus potentially enhancing their own resilience in the face of adversity.

What resonates through the following stories is not only the resiliency and inner drive to survive the challenges presented, but being able to thrive.

Through reading and reflecting on the following stories, you will learn how facing challenges allows for becoming a more empathetic nurse and a stronger person.

Pamela Delis, RN, BSN, MSN is currently undertaking a PhD program in nursing with a focus on health promotion at the University of Massachusetts/Lowell. She is a full-time faculty member for the school of nursing at Salem State University, and works part time as an RN with children with developmental disabilities. She lives in Massachusetts with her husband, dog, and two cats. Her son is at college pursuing pre-medical studies.

Reference

East, L., Jackson, D., O'Brien, L., Peters K. (2010). Storytelling: An approach that can help to develop resilience. *Journal of Nursing Research*, 17(3), 17-25.

2 REASONABLE ACCOMMODATION: LEGAL PROTECTION FOR NURSES WITH DISABILITIES

By Susan B. Matt, RN, MN, JD, PHD

Less than a quarter of a century ago, individuals with disabilities were widely considered incapable of contributing to the economy. There were no legal protections for these people in the workplace; and a nurse with a disability was rarely – if ever – heard of because most worked hard at hiding their disabilities. With the passage of the Rehabilitation Act of 1973 (Rehab Act), the climate began to change, and the Americans with Disabilities Act of 1990 (ADA) gave nurses and other workers with disabilities a weapon to fight the discriminatory practices that prevented them from obtaining and keeping employment. The 2008 amendments to the ADA, which became effective on January 1, 2009, provided clarification regarding the intent behind the original law and increased protection for people with disabilities.

The Rehab Act prohibits discrimination against individuals with any handicap by any entity receiving federal funding. Section 501 applies to the federal government; Section 503 to companies that do business with the federal government; and Section 504 to recipients of federal financial assistance. Thus, any healthcare employer receiving Medicare payments or that is in any way connected to the federal government or federal funding is covered under this law. (29 U.S.C. § 791).

Enacted to further level the playing field for people with disabilities, the ADA incorporated most of the standards established under the Rehab Act. Title I of the ADA protects individuals with disabilities in the workplace. Despite numerous attempts to narrow the protections available under these laws, the core legislative intent remains intact. Under both acts, employers are required to provide reasonable accommodation to qualified individuals with disabilities. Under the ADA, however, as in other federal antidiscrimination laws, an employer is not covered unless its

16

workforce includes "15 or more employees for each working day for each of 20 or more calendar weeks in the current or preceding calendar year" (42 U.S.C. §12111(5); Clackamas v. Wells, 2003). But employers not covered under the ADA are still required to meet this standard under the Rehab Act.

In addition to federal laws, state discrimination laws may have mandates that are different than those in the Rehab Act or ADA (Parry, 2008). Often, state laws are stronger, providing even greater protection for nurses with disabilities. It is important to learn about the protections afforded in the state where the nurse practices.

Qualified Individuals with Disabilities

The Rehab Act and Title I of the ADA were enacted to protect "qualified individuals" in the workplace (42 U.S.C. § 12101 *et seq.*; 29 U.S.C. § 791 *et seq.;* U.S. Equal Employment Opportunity Commission, 2009). But what constitutes a qualified individual?

According to the ADA definition, a qualified individual is one "who, *with or without reasonable accommodation* [italics added], can perform the essential functions of the employment position that such individual holds or desires" (42 U.S.C. § 12111(8)).

The law specifically defines "disability" with respect to an individual as:

(A) a physical or mental impairment that substantially limits one or more major life activities of such individual

(B) a record of such an impairment or

(C) being regarded as having such an impairment (42 U.S.C. § 12102(1)).

Since 1992, when the Equal Employment Opportunity Commission published its ADA Technical Assistance Manual, the U.S. Supreme Court has considered a number of cases involving employees with disabilities. Its rulings have altered the definition of the term "disability," limiting the population protected by the ADA (Sutton v. United Airlines, Inc., 1999; Murphy v. United Parcel Service, Inc., 1999). As a result of these decisions, the manual's addendum advised that "[w]hether a person has an ADA disability is determined by taking into account the positive and negative effects of mitigating measures used by the individual" (EEOC, October 2002). In practical terms, this meant that if one has little or no difficulty performing any major life activity as a result of use of a "mitigating measure," such as hearing aids or medication to control a disabling medical condition, one might not have met the first prong of the ADA's definition of an individual with a disability. In 2008, Congress passed the Americans with Disabilities Act Amendments Act (ADAAA), rejecting case law and restoring the breadth of protection intended when the original ADA was passed in 1990. The ADAAA provides that the ameliorative effects of mitigating measures should not be considered in determining whether an individual has an impairment that substantially limits a major life activity. (The ADA Amendments Act of 2008, 42 USC § 12101 note, sec. 3(4)(E)).

The original ADA relied on the Rehab Act regulations issued by the Department of Health, Education and Welfare (HEW) in 1977, which defined "physical or mental impairment" and "major life activity." Physical impairment is considered "any physiological disorder or condition, cosmetic disfigurement, or anatomical loss affecting one or more of the following body systems: neurological; musculoskeletal; special sense organs; respiratory, including speech organs; cardiovascular; reproductive, digestive, genitourinary; hemic and lymphatic; skin; and endocrine." (45 CFR § 84.3(j)(2)(i)(A) (2001)). Mental impairment is considered "any mental or psychological disorder, such as mental retardation, organic brain syndrome, emotional or mental illness, and specific learning disabilities." (45 CFR § 84.3(j)(2)(i)(B) (2001)). The HEW Rehab Act regulations provide examples of major life activities that include walking, seeing, hearing and performing manual tasks. (45 CFR 84.3(j)(2)(ii) (2001). This was expanded by the ADAAA to include the operation of "major bodily function," such as the immune system, normal cell growth, and the endocrine system. (The ADA Amendments Act of 2008, 42 USC § 12101 note, sec. 3(2)(B)).

The bottom line? For individuals to be protected by the Rehabilitation Act and the ADA, they must have a physical or mental impairment that substantially limits one or more major life activity *and* must meet the job qualifications and be able to perform the essential functions of the job *with or without reasonable accommodation.*

Reasonable Accommodation

Assuming that a nurse meets the initial criteria of the ADA, the key consideration for employment is "reasonable accommodation." For an employer to be required to provide any accommodation, the nurse must first ask for it. An employee cannot remain silent and expect the employer to bear the initial burden of identifying the need for and suggesting an appropriate accommodation (Matt, 2003). The ADA states under Title I that "reasonable accommodation" may include:

(A) making existing facilities used by employees readily accessible to and usable by individuals with disabilities and

(B) job restructuring, part-time or modified work schedules, reassignment to a vacant position, acquisition or modification of equipment or devices, appropriate adjustment or modifications of examinations, training materials or policies, the provision of qualified readers or interpreters, and other similar accommodations for individuals with disabilities. (42 U.S.C. § 12111(9)).

The reasonableness of an accommodation depends upon a common sense balancing of the costs and benefits to both employer and employee (Lyons v. Legal Aid Society, 1995). An accommodation may not be considered unreasonable merely because it requires the employer to assume more than a minimal cost or because it will cost more to obtain the same overall performance from an employee with a disability. An employer is not required to provide accommodation if it presents an "undue hardship." This is defined as requiring significant difficulty or expense when taking into consideration a number of factors specific to the covered employer's business (42 U.S.C. § 12111(10)).

How does one go about deciding where the line is between reasonable accommodation and undue hardship? With respect to equipment or structural accommodations, the cost to the employer is considered along with the overall financial resources of the employer, among other factors (42 U.S.C. § 12111(10)(B)).

If a specific situation requires reassignment to accommodate the disability, the employer is required to comply. However, the employer is not obligated to reassign the nurse to a better position than he would normally be entitled to, nor is the employer obligated to provide the accommodation the nurse requests or prefers if an alternative reasonable accommodation is offered (Henricks-Robinson v. Excel, 1997; Schmidt v. Methodist Hospital, 1996). Furthermore, seniority takes priority over disability in reassignment requests. So, if a nurse is reassigned to a "light duty" position because he cannot lift patients, but another nurse with seniority requests such reassignment, that nurse can "bump" the nurse with a disability out of the job (US Airways v. Barnett, 2002).

Under the ADA, reasonable accommodation is required in three aspects of employment:

1. to ensure equal opportunity in the application process

2. to enable a qualified individual with a disability to perform the essential functions of a job and

3. to enable a disabled employee to enjoy equal benefits and privileges of employment (EEOC, May 2002).

Examples of some acceptable accommodations in each category relevant to nurses follow.

The Application Process

The application process can be quite challenging for a nurse with a disability. Without reasonable accommodation, an opportunity may be lost due to misunderstandings. To prevent such a scenario, a nurse with a moderate hearing loss may require an assistive communication device during the interview. Let's say the applicant requests provision of a PockeTalker, a device that amplifies sound during one-on-one interactions. This meets the ADA requirement of reasonable accommodation by mitigating the effects of the applicant's hearing disability and allows him or her to effectively communicate during the interview process. Individuals with mobility challenges may require accessible physical space for interviewing. This must be provided by the potential employer to comply with the ADA.

It is important to be aware that there may be reasons directly related to a disabling condition for an employer to legitimately deny employment. One that could apply to the healthcare field has already been addressed by the courts, which have maintained that the ADA permits an employer to refuse to hire an individual with a disability because his performance on the job would endanger his own health (Chevron U.S.A. v. Echazabal, 2002).

Consider as an example a nurse with an immune deficiency who is denied employment in a facility that provides healthcare to individuals diagnosed with a variety of infections that, if contracted by the nurse, would endanger the nurse's health. In such a scenario, an employer may be legally permitted to deny employment.

Performance of Essential Functions

An employer is not obligated to decrease performance standards as an accommodation, nor is it required to provide personal use items, such as hearing aids (EEOC, January 1992). Provision of auxiliary devices and services is included in the ADA mandate. Examples of such devices and services for nurses who are deaf, hard of hearing or who have other communication-related disabilities include, but are not limited to: telecommunication devices for deaf individuals (TDDs, also referred to as TTYs) for communicating by telephone; sign language and oral interpreters (not necessarily practical in a nursing environment, but may be acceptable in an educational or other work setting); computer-assisted real-time transcription (CART) services (also may be impractical in a nursing setting); note takers for training courses and meetings; captioned training tapes; and assistive listening systems.

In a situation where a nurse cannot hear blood pressure sounds, a digital blood pressure device may be a sufficient accommodation. Technological advancement has provided medical professionals with a variety of tools to accommodate hearing disabilities, including stethoscopes that translate sounds into visual displays, permitting nurses who are hard of hearing to assess heart and lung sounds.

It may be necessary to redefine the job duties as a reasonable accommodation. An employee must be able to perform the essential functions of the job, but where it is possible to remove certain *nonessential* tasks from an employee's work requirements, it should be done.

In some nursing units, shift reports are provided using a tape recorder. These recordings are often impossible for a nurse with a hearing loss to hear and understand. As reasonable accommodation, the employer might require a face-to-face report that would allow the disabled nurse to use speech-reading skills to supplement his or her hearing.

Nurses are often expected to lift and turn patients in acute care and long-term care settings. For a nurse with physical limitations that preclude him or her from performing such tasks, it may be possible for the employer to reassign those tasks to another worker, such as a nurse's aide. This may be more readily accomplished in a larger facility with more extensive staffing than in a smaller one with minimal staff. As detailed earlier, any accommodation is not "reasonable" if it results in "undue hardship" for the employer.

Some nurses work in settings other than direct patient care. For nurses working in an office setting (i.e., telephone triage), physical changes to the workplace might be necessary. For example, a desk might be lowered to accommodate a wheelchair, or the employer might provide a nurse who is hard of hearing with an amplified telephone or a CapTel--a telephone with limited captioning capabilities that relies on a third-party captioner's participation.

Nurses with certain disabling medical conditions may require breaks at specific times to monitor blood sugar levels, self-administer medications, or avoid extreme fatigue. An employer should ensure that regularly scheduled breaks are provided as accommodation and make allowances for needed relief on an emergency basis.

Equal Benefits and Privileges of Employment

It may be necessary for an employer to make physical changes to the workplace allowing for an employee with a disability to enjoy the benefit of an employee cafeteria or break room. Such changes may include installing a ramp or lowering the sink to enable a person with a mobility impairment to enter the area and reach the sink. If the employer provides a television in the employee break room, the employer would be required to provide an infrared assistive listening device or captioning to enable a hard-of-hearing employee to enjoy the same benefit of hearing the television enjoyed by other employees.

Summary

Wading through the legal requirements of disability laws is no easy feat for the nurses requesting accommodations or for the employers who must decide whether such requests are reasonable.

The laws intend to eliminate discrimination against people with disabilities in all areas of life. Nurses with disabilities are entitled to request and receive reasonable accommodation to enable them to perform the essential functions of a job. Furthermore, they have the right to equal enjoyment of the benefits and privileges of employment. By knowing the law, nurses with disabilities can ensure that they are afforded the same opportunities available to other nurses, thereby benefiting the general population needing the care of a competent, compassionate nurse.

Susan B. Matt, PhD, JD, MN, RN, is an assistant professor at the Seattle University College of Nursing in Seattle, Washington. She is also an attorney whose practice is limited to disability law. Susan earned her PhD in nursing and her juris doctor from the University of Washington in Seattle. She earned her BSN from the College of New Rochelle in New York and a master's in neuroscience nursing from the University of Washington. Her career took her from the bedside to administration and risk management, which sparked her interest in law. A passion for disability law grew from her severe hearing loss. Her dissertation research focused on nurses with disabilities and disability climate in hospital workplaces. She lives with her husband of 37 years, the youngest of her four children and a menagerie of pets. Susan can be reached at matts@seattleu.edu.

References

29 U.S.C. § 791 *et seq.*

42 U.S.C. § 12101 *et seq.*

45 C.F.R. § 84.3 (2001, 2002).

Chevron U.S.A. Inc., Petitioner v. Mario Echazabal,536 U.S. 73, 122 S. Ct. 2045, 2002.

Clackamas Gastroenterology Associates, P.D., Petitioner v. Deborah Wells, 123 S. Ct. 1673, 2003.

Henricks-Robinson v. Excel, Case No. 94-3156 (D.C.D. Ill. 1997).

Lyons v. Legal Aid Society, 68 F.3d 1512 (2nd Cir. 1995).

Matt, S.B. (2003). Reasonable accommodation: What does the law really require?

Journal of the Association of Medical Professionals with Hearing Losses, 1(3). Retrieved on January 27, 2014 from http://www.amphl.org/articles/matt2003.pdf.

Murphy v. United Parcel Service, Inc., 527 U.S. 516 (1999).

Parry, J. (2008). *Disability discrimination law, evidence and testimony: A comprehensive reference manual for lawyers, judges and disability professionals.* Chicago, Ill: American Bar Association.

Schmidt v. Methodist Hospital, 89 F.3d 342 (7th Cir. 1996).

Sutton v. United Airlines, Inc., 527 U.S. 471 (1999).

The ADA Amendments Act of 2008, 42 USC § 12101 note.

US Airways, Inc., Petitioner v. Robert Barnett,535 U.S. 391, 122 S. Ct. 1516, 2002.

U.S. Equal Opportunity Commission (January 1992). *A technical assistance manual on the employment provisions (Title I) of the Americans with Disabilities Act.*

U.S. Equal Opportunity Commission (October 2002). *A technical assistance manual on the employment provisions (Title I) of the Americans with Disabilities Act Addendum.* Retrieved on January 27, 2014 from http://www.eeoc.gov/policy/docs/adamanual_add.html

U.S. Equal Opportunity Commission (2009). *Federal laws prohibiting job discrimination questions and answers.* Retrieved on January 27, 2014 from www.eeoc.gov/facts/qanda.html.

U.S. Equal Employment Opportunity Commission (2009). *Notice concerning The Americans With Disabilities Act (ADA) Amendments Act of 2008.* Retrieved on January 27, 2014 from www.eeoc.gov/ada/amendments_notice.html.

3 NAVIGATING THE VOCATIONAL REHABILITATION SYSTEM: NURSING FOLLOWING INJURY AND DISABILITY

By Rebecca S. Koszalinski, MS, RN, CRRN, HTL(ASCP),
PhD student

Now that disability has happened and life has changed, another challenge is before you— including many questions to answer: Can I go back to work? Can I go back to school? Or, should I go on Social Security Disability? These are difficult questions that only you can answer. Knowledge is power so you should know as much as possible before making a decision. Much of the information to follow is based on personal experience. It should be used *only* as a guide. Your journey may be different.

The good news is that state vocational rehabilitation programs can help some nurses and nursing students gain, maintain and advance employment. It is possible to navigate the vocational rehabilitation system and possibly secure financial support for equipment (e.g. amplified stethoscope) or funds for tuition for a nursing program. But you need to know the rules and understand how the system works.

Social Security Disability

You must have worked a specific amount of time and earned a specific amount of money before you can receive benefits. The rules may change, so you will need to consult your local Social Security Administration (SSA) office for current information. If you have worked a day under or received a dollar more than the rules specify, you will not qualify for benefits. If your request is refused, you can appeal, but it will take time (years for some people). No amount of yelling or screaming will hurry the process as there are others in line, so it is best to remain polite and thoughtful. It is just a matter of waiting your turn. You need to use nursing ingenuity and patience to get this done.

Also, keep in mind that if you claim Social Security Disability (SSD) you are claiming that you *cannot work in any way, shape, or form*. So, an important question to ask yourself is: "Do you want to stay home on SSD for the rest of your life?

You might want to begin by investigating what is possible for you to do other than going back to work as a staff nurse. For example, could you work from home? Could you do telephone triage? Or, work at a nurse call center? As a nurse, you have skills that may be used in other ways. For example, insurance companies may need your expertise doing chart review or processing claims.

The Department of Vocational Rehabilitation (VR) system is something to navigate *only* if there is no other alternative. If you decide to file, you will most likely be denied the first time. In my experience, it is rare that a nurse is approved quickly. You will need to appeal and the process *generally goes like the following: With the first appeal, you have 60 days from the receipt of the letter to file for reconsideration. Allow at least four to six months for a reply (calling to check on it will not speed the process but do keep track of elapsed time). If you are denied reconsideration, you then have the right to an informal hearing with an administrative judge. At this meeting, your records will be reviewed and you will have an opportunity to speak and there will be a decision made. If your case is denied following this meeting, then you have 60 days to file an appeal which will decide if you are allowed another hearing (Appeal Council). Then the case is decided (for or against you) or sent back to where you begin again.

It is a long and tedious process, so try to find a way to stay renewed and resilient. You need to be certain that you need this service and that you are not wasting your time. In other words: If this is what you choose to do then you need to be strong and certain. If you are paid for any type of service while on this benefit, you must report every penny. If you exceed the limit by the smallest amount, your case will be reviewed and benefits may cease and you will be responsible for any overpayment.

*Experiences can vary in different states.

Know Your Legal Rights Under the Americans with Disabilities Act

You need to know about the Americans with Disability Act of 1990 (ADA) including changes made by the ADA Amendments Act of 2008 (see Chapter 2). It is a tool to *attempt* to level the playing field. The ADA page is updated with monthly newsletters and cases. It can be found at http://www.ada.gov/new.htm.

Education Is Key

To any nurse with a disability, going back to school and earning an advanced degree is imperative. Advanced degrees will increase your employment options. You may be allowed to draw benefits while pursuing a degree. But you do not want to stay on the system any longer than necessary because there is an expectation that even if you are attending school, you fully intend to return to the workforce. Also, a prolonged period of time of being on benefits may cause you to fall behind on current nursing practices. And it's more difficult to find a position if you're not up to date. Theoretical knowledge is excellent, but you need to know what is currently happening at the bedside.

State Vocational Rehabilitation Programs

Your state's VR may be able to assist your return to school to become a nurse or obtain an advanced degree in nursing. If your case is solid and your track record indicates that you are a "good risk" and will complete school and then work, the VR may agree to help you. If you have an undergraduate degree, then you must be prepared to defend why you cannot work with that degree and clearly explain the career options that will open with an advanced degree.

Additional good news is that personal bias is now better controlled with the development of Policy Directive 97-04 (U.S. Department of Education, 1997). Previously, counselors had a great deal of power in deciding your ability to work and essentially offering options as they saw them. Through this directive, the practice of possibly limiting goals was overturned. You are now urged to set your own goals and VR tries to formulate ways to help you get there. Your goals have to be reasonable—so develop realistic goals.

Your state vocational rehabilitation representative most likely won't be a nurse or an expert on alternative nursing career paths. To them, a nurse is a nurse—period. That is why *you* need to *help them help you*. They can't support your case unless they understand your goals and have documentation to support the plan. Be prepared for a lack of understanding and rejections. Again, it is not personal. Justification is not based on the number of years you have worked, but on your physical condition and the probability that you will return to work if they support you.

Let negative responses fuel your next step. Don't take "no" for an answer. Turn "no" into…ok who else can I talk to? Or, what else can I do? And of course, document; document everything and keep copies. Also, be polite when speaking to government representatives. They cannot jump the queue with your case but they can make the journey less uncomfortable by listening to you and offering validation of your frustration.

Keep your goals realistic but if you find the process impossible and you feel unheard, know that you have recourse. Recourse can be found in your state's client assistant program (CAP). CAP serves these basic roles; 1) Inform and advise applicants; 2) Assist clients and applicants in obtaining services; 3) Investigate complaints about services provided; 4) Assist clients and applicants with problem resolution; 5) Assist in appeals made by counselors and; 6) Represent clients and recipients in administrative, legal or other appropriate proceedings (Disability Rights Montana).

Develop a Proposal

If you know how to develop a proposal, then write one. If you do not know how to develop a proposal, then you need to learn. The state representatives need to know that you have a plan, will follow through on the plan and return on the investment. A formal proposal should be typed (and include your personal situation, disability, previous education and work experience, and long-term goals). This will facilitate their understanding of your goals.

I wanted VR support to obtain a master's degree, so I could teach nursing. The proposal I submitted included evidence of the current shortage of nursing faculty from the National League of Nursing and American Association of Colleges of Nursing. I also included data from the U.S. Department of Labor regarding the projected need for postsecondary teachers—further evidence of employment possibilities. Advertisements for positions you will be seeking and evidence of other nurses with a disability similar to yours, who are working, should be included as well. Share journal articles, anecdotal accounts and books about nurses working with disabilities. (See Appendix C)

Ticket to Work

Using the Ticket to Work (Social Security Administration, 2010) is tricky. If you choose to use Ticket to Work, you cannot earn a penny without reporting it. So, you are allowed to work with this ticket but you are under the same rules of SSD. You cannot earn over a certain amount of money per month (consult your local office).

Misunderstanding occurs when people are unaware that the Ticket to Work means you are able to work *but* there are rules to be followed. If you exceed the income limits and do not report, it will come back to haunt you. Stating, "I did not know" is not a valid excuse and they will exact what they consider to be an overpayment from you. Keep excellent records.

For each month you report any earnings, put a copy in the mail to yourself and then do not open it when it arrives to ensure you have a valid copy with the postmarked date it was sent to the SSA office. Documentation sent to your SSA office should also be tracked with receipts. This proof is inexpensive and well worth the peace of mind of going the extra step. Be careful with what you send electronically (email) and know that everything you send goes into your file.

The Ticket to Work program is complicated. Information can be found on the Internet or from a visit to your local SSA office. The system is beautiful *when* it works. However, in any system this large, someone along the way is bound to drop the ball.

Final Thoughts and Affirmations

This is not what you expected when you became a nurse. However, remember that you weathered school and the nursing boards to become a nurse, so you have the ability to rise above this challenge. Some people will try to assist while others will caution against trying to make lemonade out of a lemon situation.

I traveled this road after being severely injured as a gymnast. Over the years, I have found that some nurses with disabilities get through this system and others continue to struggle. People who go into nursing are usually self-starters and full of innovation. Use that innovation to return to school, become a nurse educator or find a new dream. Know that the dream is within you—not within the government representative working with your case.

Remember people are cheering for you— so take heart.

You've gotten this far … travel on…

Building Resilience

Work *with* your state Vocational Rehabilitation program

Extend your hand with introductions

Turn "no" into inspiring your next step

Present an organized proposal

Be professional

Follow up

Be proactive but not a pest

Rebecca S. Koszalinski, RN, MS, CRRN graduated from University of Wisconsin-Oshkosh. She earned her MS at Florida Atlantic University. Rebecca is currently a doctoral student and faculty member at Florida Atlantic University's Christine E. Lynn College of Nursing. She has lower limb lymphedema and uses a forearm crutch. She can be reached at sbbk4him@bellsouth.net.

References

Disability Rights Montana. *Client assistance program.* Retrieved on January 27, 2014 from http://disabilityrightsmt.org/janda3/inner.php?PageID=63

Department of Justice. *ADA Homepage.* Retrieved January 27, 2014 from http://www.ada.gov/

Division of Vocational Rehabilitation (2011). *Handbook of Services: Your Guide to Employment.* Tallahassee: Department of Vocational Rehabilitation. Retrieved on January 27, 2014 from http://www.rehabworks.org/docs/HandbookofServices.txt

Social Security Administration. *Ticket to work.* Retrieved January 27, 2014 from https://yourtickettowork.com/web/ttw/en-about-ticket-to-work

U.S. Department of Education, Office of Special Education and Rehabilitative Services (1997). *Policy Directive 97-04.* Retrieved on January 27, 2014 from http://www2.ed.gov/offices/OSERS/RSA/guidance/PD-97-04.pdf

Suggested Reading

Huffman, L. & Strechay, J. (2010). Insider Tips for Getting the Most from Vocational Rehabilitation. *AFB Access World Magazine*, 11 (6). Retrieved on January 27, 2014 from

http://www.afb.org/afbpress/pub.asp?DocID=aw110602

COMMENTARY

By Jim Marks, BA

The author's emphasis on documenting and approaching vocational rehabilitation as a well-informed and self-reliant person hits the mark exceptionally well. I think many individuals with disabilities approach service providers as though the service providers have all the answers. It's better to look on service providers as partners, and this chapter does that well. After all, people with disabilities don't have to live down to the stereotype of the passive, helpless individual. We can and should direct our services just as the author recommends. Nice job!

The vocational goal drives the vocational rehabilitation process. The Rehabilitation Act, its regulations, and administrative rules clearly give individuals with disabilities a great deal of control in deciding what that vocational goal should be. In its policy directive 97-04, the Rehabilitation Services Administration overturned previous practices that gave the vocational rehabilitation counselor strong powers to determine whether a goal was suitable or reasonable for a client. Now, thanks to that 1997 Policy Directive and amendments to the Rehabilitation Act itself, individuals with disabilities may have vocational goals that are "consistent with their strengths, resources, priorities, concerns, abilities, and capabilities."

Of course, practice may stray from policy, regulations, and the law. Some counselors may cling to outdated practices. This is why it is so important to include information about due process in vocational rehabilitation.

Each state must offer a CAP, and its purpose is to assist individuals with disabilities who disagree with decisions made by the vocational rehabilitation agency. Essentially, when a vocational rehabilitation counselor says, "no," it might not actually mean "no" thanks to these strong appeals systems.

Jim Marks, BA, is the director of disability transitions services for the state of Montana

Department of Public Health and Human Services. He administers several programs including vocational rehabilitation, blind and low vision and independent living services. He can be reached at jimmarks@mt.gov.

References

Rehabilitation Services Administration, US Dept. of Education. http://www2.ed.gov/about/offices/list/osers/rsa/index.html

Client Assistance Program, Rehabilitation Services Administration

http://www2.ed.gov/programs/rsacap/index.html

4 TAKING THE FIRST STEP: NURSING WITH SACRAL AGENESIS

By Susie Cutino Pratt MSN, MPS, BSN, RN

Having a physical disability as a nurse can be an everyday struggle. I often speak to student nurses who question, even doubt, their potential as nurses because of their own physical issues. I want to empower more student nurses to find their place in the most rewarding career of a lifetime— empower them just like my mother empowered me.

"When God created you he did not finish his product. He gave you problems that sometimes I blame myself for. I often wonder do you curse me for having you? Are you angry at me?"

"This may sound strange coming from your mother but I have always carried this feeling within me. All the years of your growing up, I prayed. We went to so many different doctors, always looking for the perfect answer for you. But to no avail, every new method of doing a new procedure we tired. …The problem with you brought daddy and I together--as close as anyone could be. All we lived for was for you--to make you stronger health wise and mentally. You grew into a beautiful young woman with great traits toward people and a lot of heart. School was never easy for you but you worked at it until you got what you wanted. Your Dad and I tried talking you out of nursing, feeling it was too hard a life for you, but you fought us proudly and became a nurse, which was one of the happiest moments in my life."

My mother wrote these words in 1996. I only read the title, "One Incomplete Child," and put the letter away for another day. Since then, both my parents passed away.

I write about this letter today because it has more meaning now. While working on a paper for a nursing theory class, "The Theory of Chronic Sorrow," my eyes were opened. The theory explains how parents of children who have a physical or mental disability struggle to cope with loss of a "perfect child" (Eakes, Burke, Hainsworth, 1998). My mom struggled all of her adult life with her loss of the perfect child. I was the child with the physical disability. She titled her letter "One Incomplete Child," which explains her own chronic sorrow she experienced having me. Sadly, we never had a chance to talk about the letter before she died. I never knew she blamed herself for my condition. We were so close and yet she never discussed her feelings. Her feeling of considering me being an incomplete child was so overwhelming when I read the letter, I cried.

A Neural Tube Defect

When I was born, my parents were told that I had a congenital defect called spina bifida. Later, through genetic counseling, I was told my true diagnosis was caudal regression anomaly, specifically sacral agenesis. This is a neural tube defect, which prevents the development of a sacrum or coccyx. Having no sacrum or coccyx caused weakness of my lower extremities. My mom wrote how hard it was for her and my dad to raise a child with physical disabilities. I had many physical problems growing up, but the encouragement and reassurance from the people around me gave me the will to go on.

Besides my parents, nurses gave me lots of encouragement. I was always in and out of hospitals for one reason or another but the nurses at the hospital were always compassionate, supportive and reassuring. I think this is the reason I so wanted to become a nurse. To give encouragement, support and inspiration to others who have physical disabilities. After reading the letter, I now know how hard it was for my parents to understand why I pursued a nursing career.

I never considered myself "One Incomplete Child", as my mom wrote, until I went to college. Until then, I was always part of the "normal" world. A professor at Long Island University developed a program for students with disabilities. Meeting the requirements, I was accepted to the program. The program was set up to give the students academic support and accommodations for their disability. Students had cerebral palsy, spina bifida and many other disabilities, but each one had the same goal in mind: to go to college.

When I told a professor that I wanted to become a nurse, he made an appointment for me to meet with the director of the nursing department. At the end of the interview, I was shocked when the director asked me to walk for her. This was well before the American with Disabilities Act was passed. Apparently, she wanted to see if I could walk fast enough to help someone in an emergency.

Inspiration to Succeed

For the first time in my life, I felt like I *was* an "incomplete child." This feeling of incompleteness made me more determined to become a nurse. It gave me greater strength and determination to follow my dream. I overcame many obstacles in my life but each one made me stronger and more confident in my professional nursing career. This made me even more determined to continue my education and become a nurse educator.

I've been a nurse for more than 30 years. Over the years, I have held many different positions. When I interviewed for jobs, management never questioned me about whether or not I could handle the physical demands of the position. Every opportunity seemed to open a door for another successful step in my nursing career path. Currently, I teach practical nursing students, a position I have held for 10 years.

I look back now on my remarkable career and realize that the most important step was the one I took some 30 years ago for the director of Long Island University's Nursing School.

Building Resilience

Take the first step

Turn "incomplete" feelings into strength and determination

Follow your dream

Seize every opportunity as a new door opening

Susie Cutino Pratt BSN, MPS, RN is an instructor in the practical nursing program at Lincoln Technical Institute in New Britain, Connecticut. She received her MSN from the University of Hartford. Susie can be reached at cutino13@sbcglobal.net.

Reference

Eakes, G., Burke, M. & Hainsworth, M. (1998). Middle-range theory of chronic sorrow. *Journal of Nursing Scholarship, 30*(2), 179–184.

COMMENTARY

By Susan E. Fleming PhD, RN, Perinatal CNS

What a beautiful story of how one young woman overcame many obstacles in order to achieve her goal of becoming a nurse, in spite of her limitations being born with spina bifida. She shares her compelling story of how she found her mother's letter, titled "One Incomplete Child". She recognized that this was her mother's perception related to her own sorrow and perhaps even her own concealed guilt. In an effort to protect her from the harsh reality of pursuing a career in a physically demanding profession of nursing, her parents discouraged her. As she progressed through the educational system, she found the system to be unwelcoming. Relentlessly, she proceeds and becomes a nurse—taking full ownership of her success.

I can relate to this young woman being born with a disability. I was born without my left hand, and became a nurse by navigating my way through an unwelcoming educational system. However, my mother was extremely supportive of me throughout my journey of desiring and then pursuing to become a nurse. The influence of nurses helped as well. "I fondly remember the gift of visionary hope that the nurses and other health team members gave to me and my mother. Their vision of my success empowered us and gave us strength" (Fleming, 2007 p. 164).

Instilling Independence

My mother, a kindergarten teacher, banned any effort by others to offer extra help for me. When I was three years old, our neighbors rushed to help me when I fell, and my mother rebuked their actions by saying, "Stop that, how will she ever learn to take care of herself if you over compensate for her?" As she had counseled my siblings who did not have limitations, she maintained that I could pursue any career I desired, as long as I was willing to work. My mother would have never dreamed of calling me an incomplete child.

In retrospect, I wonder if she felt she would have had to take ownership of my birth defect, if she did. I once asked her if she ever felt guilty, she callously stated, "Of course not, I never did anything wrong." As a mother of seven, I find that statement odd. In my early years as a mother, I reveled with my children's success and mourned with their failures. It took many years for me to recognize that they were their own persons responsible for their own fate.

"Nursing educators need to be open to admission of more students with disabilities. All nurses, educators and administrators can make a difference in the success of students and their perceptions of themselves as a valued member of the nursing team. We need to encourage all nursing students to know their strengths and build on them." Fleming & Maheady (2004, p.536.) Nurse educators and administrators need to recognize the gifts that students and nurses with disabilities bring to practice.

Nurses caring for children with disabilities need to offer gifts of visionary hope. Regardless of parental feelings and attitudes, children with disabilities appear to come preloaded with their own innate strength— that allows them to conquer the cruelties of this world and move forward. And when faced with obstacles, they can challenge the status quo and "reinvent" themselves so they can have the life they've dreamed of having. "The child could even grow up to be a nurse" (Fleming & Maheady, 2004, p.536).

Susan E. Fleming PhD, RN, Perinatal CNS, is an assistant professor at Washington State University College of Nursing. Dr. Fleming has written many articles about nurses and nursing students with disabilities. She has also developed audiovisual training materials for nurses and nursing students with disabilities learning nursing skills. Dr. Fleming wrote a book about her grandmother called *Alice Ada Wood Ellis: Seattle Pioneer Midwife, Nurse, & Mother to All* (2014*). She is a board member of* www.ExceptionalNurse.com *and can be reached at* susan.fleming@email.wsu.edu.

References

Fleming, S.E. (2007). Hope for parents of newborns with disabilities. *Journal of Christian Nursing*, 24 (3), 164.

Fleming, S., & Maheady, D. (2004). Empowering Persons with Disabilities. *AWHONN Lifelines*, 8 (6), 534-537.

5 AIN'T NO MOUNTAIN HIGH ENOUGH: PATHS TO SUCCESS FOR NURSES WITH LEARNING DISABILITIES

By Tino Plank, RN, MS

The song, "Ain't No Mountain High Enough" is about having the determination to overcome obstacles and be with the one you love. For me, this song became an inspiration to face my learning challenges in order to do what I love. I was simply determined not to let my disabilities, or other people's reactions to them dampen my enthusiasm for learning—or keep me from pursuing a career in nursing. Building a network of support and facing the seemingly mountainous challenges—head on—were keys to my success.

From an early age, teachers always remarked that I was an underachieving student. What I heard and internalized was they thought I wasn't trying hard enough, or I wasn't smart enough to get better grades. What I understand now is that my then-undiagnosed learning disabilities affected my ability to process information. My grades and my level of class participation were not in any way a reflection of my ability to learn, my talents, or my intelligence.

As an adult, I worked as a hospice grief counselor. As I listened to my clients and their families, I frequently heard about something they wished they had done, or wished their loved one had experienced. Many times, these postponed dreams centered on a long-deferred educational or career goal. After years of hearing this repeated theme of regret, I realized that I needed to explore my own regrets.

What scared me most weren't the long hours of studying that lay ahead—I actually love learning new things—it was that I'm a different kind of learner. Fortunately, the community college where I took my prerequisite courses had an excellent disability services department. The staff helped me get tested, and they documented my learning style so that I could receive accommodations. I also discovered the importance of self-advocacy in challenging prejudices about the invisible nature of my disabilities.

Learning Disabilities

Sadly, the label of *learning disabled* is often mistakenly associated with diminished intelligence. As a result, an unfortunate stigma is attached to having learning disabilities. In fact, many people with learning disabilities have a higher than average IQ—they just process information differently and may not flourish in the standard learning environment.

The Individuals with Disabilities Education Act (IDEA) defines a learning disability as "a disorder in one or more of the basic psychological processes involved in understanding or in using language, spoken or written, which disorder may manifest itself in the imperfect ability to listen, think, speak, read, write, spell, or do mathematical calculations" (www.ldonline.org).

While it is commonly understood that people often develop certain adaptations to compensate for losses or impairments—such as a person who learns to visually "read" lips to compensate for a hearing loss—not everyone recognizes the compensations and adaptations that people with learning disabilities use to process information in a classroom or work environment. Unlike a physical or sensory disability, learning disabilities are not outwardly visible, and people may make assumptions about what they perceive as distracted, lazy, or shy behaviors. This is why it is imperative to assess suspected disabilities and get the results documented. There is a tremendous amount of assistance and support available through schools, state departments of vocational rehabilitation, and community agencies. These resources can also provide the social support needed to combat the isolation and alienation so often associated with having a disability.

Tips and Tools

One source of support may come from looking at the lives and accomplishments of famous people with learning disabilities. Some well-known people with learning disabilities and/or ADHD include: former Vice President Nelson Rockefeller; renowned computer engineer and inventor William Hewlett; actress and comedian Whoopi Goldberg; and business leader Charles Schwab (www.greatschools.net).

While it can be inspiring to look at the achievements of other people with learning disabilities, the development of your own self-advocacy skills is essential! Self-advocacy is being able to clearly communicate your needs to others. This involves the internal process of assessing your abilities, and adaptability to determine what sort of assistance you need to fully accomplish what you want. Remember that learning disabilities tend to be invisible. Therefore, you need to know what you can do (and how you can do it) in order to educate others so they can support you.

A great self-advocacy tool I learned from an academic counselor was to create what he called a "Learning Bio." For anyone who is not comfortable speaking to an instructor (or employer) about their learning disability, this written format can be a great help. By using a learning bio, you can effectively demonstrate your desire to learn *and* inform the reader that you need assistance. Here is an example of a learning bio I used in school:

STUDENT LEARNING BIO

Tino Plank, Pre-Nursing Student

Dear_____:

My name is Tino Plank, and I'm in the process of completing my nursing school pre-requisites. At the suggestion of my academic counselor, Bill Jones, I've put together this "learning bio" as a way to introduce myself, my scholastic goals, and my learning disabilities.

I already have a B.S. degree, which I completed in 1980. However, at that time, I struggled in many of my core science classes because I didn't realize that I had learning disabilities that impacted my capacity to process the material I was studying. Specifically, I have auditory and visual processing deficits and dyslexia/ADD characteristics that slow down the way I integrate information.

I always wanted to continue my science education, but had been intimidated by the testing challenges from my undergraduate days. Fortunately, I've been through the learning skills assessment offered by Student Supportive Services, and with their guidance and support, we've worked out learning/testing accommodations that have improved my ability to learn and retain information.

I look forward to learning from you this semester and working with you to incorporate my accommodations into the classroom.

Sincerely,

Tino Plank

The counselor who suggested the learning bio was an academic counselor. He had a learning disability and was a strong advocate for accommodations. The disabilities staff was extremely supportive (and in turn, supported by the administration).

When I entered nursing school, I was direct in letting the program director and my instructors know about my disabilities. I received accommodations that included extended time on tests and a reduced distraction environment for test taking. My instructors were very supportive. In addition, the Sonoma State University disabilities services office was instrumental in starting a campus chapter of Delta Alpha Pi (an honor society for students with disabilities). In my mind, this action demonstrated to the larger university community that disabilities (including learning disabilities) did not exclude students from achieving academic honors.

I also developed an ability/adaptability assessment tool after watching classmates with physical disabilities compensate for impairments in one muscle group by using another, stronger group of muscles. In my own case, I use certain cognitive strengths to support my weaker areas.

An ability/adaptability assessment gives me the opportunity to see what my strengths, weaknesses, and possible adaptations are. I'm a very visual and kinesthetic learner, so I created something to gauge my relative ability for certain cognitive functions (like reading, doing math calculations, and organizing my thoughts). I draw a horizontal line as a zero-to-10 scale and rate my ability for a certain function with an "X" along the line. Then, I'll look at the other ratings to see if I have a stronger score in another function. Finally, I assess if I can adapt the stronger function to compensate for the weaker one. Here's a simple assessment that I might use to address my distractibility.

Ability/Adaptability Assessment for Distractibility	
Cognitive Function	Weak - Strong Scale
Visual Attention to Detail	0_____X
Auditory Concentration	0_____X_____

Using the assessment above, I know I'm distractible in a noisy environment, but I also know I have strong attention to detail. Therefore, I adapt by visually breaking a task into steps, and then making a detailed list to keep myself focused when I have multiple things to do. And like many people with learning disabilities, I was multi-tasking *way* before that term was coined. You've probably got a number of adaptations that you already use to manage your personal and work life. Write them down and see if this stimulates ideas on how to use your own abilities and adaptations to compensate for areas where you aren't quite as capable.

I also found that observing and interacting with other disabled learners was very helpful. You can do a lot of skill building by sharing ideas in social groups related to disabilities—even groups online. In addition, there is a psychological boost to being with others who can relate to your struggles. Let's face it, being perceived as different can be stressful, but being understood by others can help you cope.

If you are already a nurse, you can use these strategies to connect with a mentor or with the nurse educator and the charge nurse where you work. Just as it is important working with instructors in nursing school, it is equally important to work with employers to let them know what sort of accommodations you need. When you show an interest in becoming a better nurse, any worthwhile employer should work to support you. Besides, if you have done your ability/adaptability assessment, you can clearly discuss both your areas of strength and challenges.

Treating Your Disability

As nurses, we've all seen clients benefit from certain medications. I've heard from people who have had great results from drugs such as Ritalin, Adderall and Provigil. Similarly, I've heard from people who have gained tremendous benefits through counseling, such as cognitive behavioral therapy. However, I've also heard from other people with learning disabilities who found that counseling was ineffective or that drug side effects were worse than the symptoms they were trying to treat. For such people, focusing practices such as meditation or self-hypnosis may help with distractibility and other learning challenges. Sometimes, it can take a combination of treatments; therefore, consulting a specialist can help you treat or cope with your disability.

Nursing with Learning Disabilities

While nursing with learning disabilities can be challenging, you will likely have a surprising number of valuable abilities. It is a real no-brainer that empathy helps build a strong nurse-client relationship. Whether it's with an elderly stroke patient's inability to do activities of daily living, or an infant whose immature immune system is struggling to fight off an infection, you share a similar experience with them. Clients are in your care because they have lost some level of ability due to trauma or illness. The insights you've gathered from your own struggles and adaptations can give you great insight about how to support and comfort your clients.

In addition, one of the nursing core responsibilities is to be a client advocate. I strongly believe that another core responsibility of nurses is to develop self-advocacy skills. Becoming a strong self-advocate makes you a better client advocate. Likewise, becoming a strong client advocate allows you to develop better interpersonal boundaries and other self-care strategies. This has been a win-win skill set for me.

Using technology to compensate for a disability can be a great support strategy. After years of resisting buying a personal digital assistant (PDA), I finally got one. Now that I've gotten used to it, I can't imagine being without it. With all the healthcare-specific applications that are available for PDAs, this has become a vital way for me to organize my day. With less to keep track of in my head, I'm better focused on caring for clients.

Another great tool to help me manage my learning disabilities in the clinical setting has been using a SBAR (Situation-Background-Assessment-Recommendation) communication sheet to organize my thoughts during shift handoffs or during calls to physicians and referral sources. You can download a free copy from the Institute for Healthcare Improvement website: www.IHI.org.

Examples of workplace accommodations that I ask for are a quiet place to chart, and not having my workflow pattern disrupted, if possible. While the acute care environment isn't particularly quiet or even-paced, I've always been able to have my needs accommodated to some degree. Since I've been working in a hospital that doesn't have electronic charting, I try to chart in the client's room, which is usually quieter than the nurse's station. The information is fresh in my head, and I avoid the wasted time of taking notes and then transcribing them into the chart later.

Sometimes your accommodation might be requesting a transfer to another unit or position. For me, the emergency department would not be a good work environment, whereas an OR or a PACU unit would be much more suitable. Depending on your type of learning disability, an outpatient clinic or community health setting might be the best place to work. One of the great things about the field of nursing is that there are so many different opportunities.

Also, if your disabilities are triggered or worsened by physical and/or emotional fatigue make sure that you build self-care into your workflow. I recall being so concerned about what other nurses would think about my learning disabilities that I worked extra hard to prove a point, and I was exhausted. I follow a basic routine of getting at least eight hours of sleep a night, eating balanced meals and snacks, staying hydrated and exercising for at least 30 minutes a day. Part of my self-care routine also includes limiting (to the extent I can control it) unnecessary stimuli such as noise and intense light. Now I realize that I provide better care when I've taken care of myself.

A Reminder for Educators and Managers

Creative thinking, adaptability, advocacy, and empathy are some of the many attributes that nurses with learning disabilities have and can develop to enhance patient care. When nurse educators and nurse managers understand that disability doesn't necessarily mean less ability, they can create an environment that welcomes diverse ideas. For example, students or nurses with learning disabilities bring a different way of thinking and problem solving to the classroom or workplace. Their innate ability to think outside the box can lead to innovations that benefit everyone.

Managers can support nurses with learning disabilities by allowing accommodations that will make them more efficient and better able to provide quality client care. All nurses (with disabilities or not) have certain strengths and weaknesses, so using the ability/adaptability assessment can help identify appropriate adaptations in workflow processes for everyone.

As educators and managers, it is important to engage nurses with learning disabilities using their preferred learning style (visual, auditory, or kinesthetic). Just as we've learned to improve care by using a patient-centered approach, communication, and productivity can be enhanced using educational approaches that are student-or employee-centered. For example, if you know that a nurse has an auditory processing problem or is a visual learner, you will likely improve communication and job performance by giving written rather than oral instructions.

It took me a long time to appreciate my different adaptations and the resulting aptitudes they brought to school and work environments. In school, I had to listen very carefully to understand what my instructors were teaching. Now I see that this has translated into a heightened ability to listen attentively. Similarly, I developed a keen focus on details, because I always got tripped-up on the finer points of written tests. Ultimately, it was these same adaptations—my keen focus and attentive listening—that helped me become an honors student.

Today, these same skills are invaluable in my nursing practice and in the healthcare environment, where outcomes-based assessments and accurate charting are critical measures of effective patient care. Now my "disabilities" help me key in on subtle signs and symptoms in my clients, and listen attentively to their concerns.

In addition, my personal struggles and triumphs help me relate to the challenges that patients face. I recognize and relate to their desire and determination to heal. My disabilities have given me greater empathy and compassion for the people I care for. Having overcome stigmas and championed my own rights, I am a more powerful advocate for my patients.

Lastly, always keep in mind the benefits of your disability, and the positive influence you can have on clients and families. I wish you all the best.

Tino Plank has masters' degrees in nursing and multicultural spirituality. He is Admissions Manager for Hospice of Santa Cruz County, CA, and Adjunct Instructor for Sonoma State University's nursing department. He is a member of Sigma Theta Tau and Delta Alpha Pi honors societies. Tino also serves as a mentor for nurses with learning disabilities through www.ExceptionalNurse.com. Through his own experience and education, he provides a structure of strength and hope for patients and families as they face uncertainty and change. Likewise, he uses his artistic and spiritual training to explore the nuanced edges of the nurse/client interrelationship. He can be reached at tinoplank@emovere.com.

Building Resilience

Build a network of support

Learn from others who have blazed the trail

Identify your strengths and weaknesses

Help others help you

Create a learning/working bio

Share a summary of your accommodation needs

Take care of yourself

Use technology to your advantage

Suggested Reading

Atkinson, D., Boulter, P., Pointu, A., Thomas, B., & Moulster, G. (2010). Learning disability nursing: How to refocus the profession. *Learning Disability Practice, 13* (1), 18-21.

Children and Adults with Attention-Deficit/Hyperactivity Disorder: http://www.chadd.org/

Cowen, M. (2010). Dyslexia, dyspraxia, dyscalculia: A toolkit for nursing staff. *Royal College of Nursing.* Retrieved on January 13, 2014 from http://www.nottingham.ac.uk/studentservices/documents/rcn---dyslexiadyspraxiadyscalculia---toolkit-for-nursing-staff.pdf

Evans, W. (2013). Learn and support. *WIN, 21*(7), 24-25. Retrieved on January 13, 2014 at http://www.inmo.ie/tempDocs/Dyslexia_PAGE24AND25sep13.pdf.

George Washington University's Heath Resource Center: http://www.heath.gwu.edu/

Learning Disabilities Association of America: http://www.ldanatl.org/

LD Online: http://www.ldonline.org/

LD Pride: http://www.ldpride.net/

Learning Ally www.learningally.org

McConkey, R, & Truesdale, M. (2000). Reactions of nurses and therapists in mainstream health services to contact with people who have learning disabilities.

Journal of Advanced Nursing, 32(1), 158-63.

National Center for Learning Disabilities: http://www.ncld.org/

National Institute for Literacy: http://www.nifl.gov/

Nurse with dyslexia refuses to let reading problems stand in her way: http://www.youtube.com/watch?v=p1IiajxUIf0

Selekman, J., & Selekman, J. (2002). Updates & kidbits. Learning disabilities: a diagnosis ignored by nurses. *Pediatric Nursing, 28*(6), 630-632.

Slevin, E.,& Sines, D. (1996). Attitudes of nurses in a general hospital towards people with learning disabilities: influences of contact, and graduate-non-graduate status, a comparative study. *Journal of Advanced Nursing, 24*(6), 1116-26.

Sugg, T. (2011, February/March). Nursing success in the face of dyslexia. National Student Nurses Association Imprint Magazine, 46-47/50. Retrieved on January 27, 2014 at

http://viewer.zmags.com/publication/0f66ab6d?page=46&p8900=4842#/0f66ab6d/46

The International Dyslexia Association: http://www.interdys.org/

U.S. Department of Education: http://www.ed.gov/

COMMENTARY

By Katherine M. Kolanko, RN, PhD

Tino Plank's narrative of his experience as a person with a learning disability (LD) illustrates several important points. Most individuals with LD are not diagnosed as children. Commonly, young girls with learning disabilities are identified as under-achievers, lazy, day dreamers, sweet, quiet and "hard workers," or just not "… the brightest crayon in the box…" Because girls tend not to be a behavior problem in the classroom, their minimal achievement is overlooked. Boys, on the other hand, sometimes tend to exhibit behavior problems that are hard to manage in the classroom, such as speaking when not called on, finishing other peoples' sentences, disruptive behavior, and acting as the class clown. Since boys' issues are identified earlier, they may be referred for evaluation earlier.

Careful evaluation of the student by a licensed educational psychologist is critical to establishing the diagnosis of LD and identifying appropriate accommodations. Looking at the overall student picture or story is helpful for faculty to understand student needs. One of the most helpful strategies for faculty members to understand a student's learning needs is to ask the student to tell their personal stories, especially past learning successes or challenges. Self-motivation is an important predictor of success as well as self-assessment. For example, asking: What does Tino know about how he learns? How did Tino learn to be a grief counselor? What does he do well in his daily life? How did he learn to be successful in his daily life and career?

Finding the right college is also a key to success. If a candidate for admission discloses an LD or suspects this is a problem, a referral to services within the college designed to meet needs of all students with disabilities should be initiated. Academic institutions have policies for current evaluations, documentation, and prescription for accommodations to help the student to be successful. The college Tino entered for his nursing degree was well suited to meet the needs of students with disabilities (Kolanko, 2003).

Misconceptions of LDs

Unfortunately, most college and university faculties have limited knowledge about learning disabilities. Faculty members in and outside of nursing have many misconceptions—that include that students with LD have sub-average intellectual functioning. Those with language disabilities **cannot** read, write, spell, or can **only** just transpose letters and numbers (commonly called dyslexia). Other misconceptions include that students with math disabilities are unable to perform any math; students with LD are all the same, and students with any disability have no place in nursing or college (Brooke, 1999; Gilmore and Bose, 2005; and Kolanko, 2003).

LD is a processing difficulty. Language (reading, information processing, and writing), mathematics processing, executive functioning, and social processing are just a few manifestations of the problem. Approximately one-third of all people with learning disabilities have Attention Deficit Hyperactive Disorder (ADHD). Also, both students with LD and/or ADHD tend to have higher levels of anxiety disorders. Working with a specialist can support the individual's learning. Organizational skills and time management techniques as well as a structured environment can augment learning (Ijiri and Kudzma, 2000; and Kolanko, 2003).

Lack of knowledge on the part of college and university faculty is no excuse for not providing accommodations for students with LD. Academic institutions have a legal responsibility to follow the disability-related federal and state laws. And faculty members have a responsibility to assure a student with a disability has an environment that supports learning and success. We speak about a just culture in our healthcare organizations and we need to do the same in our educational institutions. All departments need to provide support for students with disabilities. For example, students with learning disabilities may take a reduced credit load. What does that do to the student's ability to live in dorm housing (which might be restricted to full time students)? Can students get course syllabi and learning tools (textbooks, handouts, etc.) before the semester begins so that they can prepare for classes during breaks? How will reduced loads influence financial aid (Kolanko, 2003)?

A Challenge or an Opportunity?

Tino is right when he asserts that being proactive and looking at learning disabilities (LD) as an opportunity rather than an obstacle is the right ingredient to success. Metacognition is a key to success for all college students. So the more a student with LD is able to know what strategies help them to learn and noticing when learning is breaking down, the more successful a student can be. Tino illustrates that self-regulating his learning for different subjects, being adaptable with strategies, and increasing his repertoire of learning strategies are important tools in the student's arsenal for learning success.

Breaking a task down into micro-units, using prompts, and assistive technology can help all students. We all do this whether we realize it or not (Brandt and Alwin, 2012; Kolanko, 2003). As nurses we develop sliding scale charts for delivering different dosages of IV medications, write laboratory results on our hands, and enter prompts into our iPods to be on time for medications and treatments (Kolanko, 2003; and McCleary-Jones, 2008).

Understanding deficits in social processing or lack of social skill learning is more common in college students today. Developing a network of support is important to all students with disabilities. Students with LD tend to be individual rather than group learners. But this characteristic sometimes isolates the student. Finding ways to integrate them into study groups, peer tutoring, or group discussions may help to increase the comfort level of group work and as nurses with supportive staff (Brooke, 1999). The student feels at ease and can see the group as a support rather than a source of stress.

When students with LDs learn to micro-unit (break information down into its smallest units), use various learning strategies and are provided more time, they can see the relevance of these techniques for patient care. Nurses with LD are uniquely prepared to care for patients who have the same needs. Upon learning of their LD, students report reactions of grief and loss as they see themselves as a person with a disability and not "a normal person." Helping them to self- advocate, learn success strategies, and referrals to specialists can support their needs. It should be emphasized that this is something they can help patients do for themselves as well (Kolanko, 2003). Tino found that having a learning disability can be an uncommon gift.

Case Example

A nurse educator writes: "I think a dyslexic nurse is an 'accident waiting to happen.' What will be the legal defense if he or she transposes some numbers on a medication order, such as, instead of seeing '0.5mg' she sees it as '50mg'—and she kills the patient as a result. An employer could be sued that knowingly hired a person with dyslexia and allowed her to read medication orders and then administer them."

Nurse educators face the awesome task of preparing safe and competent nurses. One of the skills considered most critical in nursing care is the safe administration of medications. So we build in safeguards around administration of medications to help the student learn this skill. These safeguards include mathematic skills, knowledge of the medication being prescribed (dosage range, usual dosage for the condition being treated, and knowledge of the medications actions, etc.), and when and how the medication is to be administered. Checks and double checks are completed by the nurse transcribing the order and the pharmacist filling the prescription, and ultimately, by the nurse giving the medication (whether it is the transcribing nurse or not).

We have medication calculation tests built into our curriculums. Many schools have math tests several times throughout their program of study. With due diligence on the part of educators, programs can graduate a nurse prepared to practice nursing safely, whether or not they have a disability.

If a nurse has dyslexia, this does not mean that every time she sees two numbers on an order, she automatically transposes them. Learning to live with a disability includes building in your own safeguards to achieve the level of competence needed. For example, current guidelines speak to the importance of the prescriber using a zero before a decimal point if there is not a whole number in the dosage being prescribed. The physician writing 0.5 mg for the dosage is an example of this. This method should cue the nurse to interpret the dosage correctly. Knowing the usual dosage range of this medication should also cue the nurse to an accurate interpretation of the prescription. The more the nurse practices nursing, the more capable he or she should become in detecting aberrations in dosage orders. If unsure, the nurse should always check dosage orders including pill identification.

Today, there are hand-held assistive devices for quick access to unfamiliar medications. Electronic records and computerized order forms can have built-in safeguards as well. Nurses should lobby their employers for software programs that can help them do their job well. Assistive devices such as talking calculators and hand-held scanning pens that will read for the nurse are readily available. With scanners, the nurse uses both sight and hearing to read the order, which greatly augments safety for a nurse with dyslexia (Kolanko, 2003; and Sharpe, Johnson, Izzo, & Murray, 2005).

The literature shows that the leading causes of nursing medication errors are due primarily to exhaustion and interruptions. There should be a thorough understanding of the root cause of each medication error (Hewitt, 2010). Is this a systemic or an individual problem? The nurse is accountable for his or her actions whether or not the nurse has a disability. The organization is accountable for providing the environment so care provided is safe. Liability from the courts' point of view would look at the probable cause of each specific error. Placing of liability is a legal matter for the courts.

Tino took a proactive approach concerning self-disclosure of his learning disability. Employers are prohibited from asking the job applicant of their status concerning a disability on an application or during an interview. After a job is offered, if the applicant wishes to disclose his or her disability, that is their choice. Employers are mandated to provide reasonable accommodations requested by the employee. Failure to provide accommodations puts the administrator at risk for a discrimination lawsuit and/or formal complaint with the Equal Employment Opportunity Commission (EEOC) on both the state and federal level. Lawsuits are costly and personal fines for discrimination can be levied on individual persons as well.

Public records of malpractice lawsuits against nurses with disabilities or their employers are not easily accessible. There is a paucity of literature available concerning long-term safety issues and overall achievement of registered nurses with disabilities. Most information is anecdotal. Further research is needed in the area of nurses and disabilities, particularly their long-term success.

Dr. Kolanko is a full professor at Franciscan University of Steubenville, Steubenville, OH. She is a nurse educator with 42 years' experience in graduate and undergraduate education. Her dissertation "A collective case study of nursing students with learning disabilities" is available through Dissertation Abstracts. She can be reached kkolanko@franciscan.edu.

References

Brandt, A. & Alwin, J. (2012). Assistive technology outcomes research: Contributions to evidence-based assistive technology practice. *Technology & Disability, 24*(1), 5-7.

Brooke, V. (1999). It's up to us: Practice and attitudes cannot be legislated. *Journal of Vocational Rehabilitation, 12*(1), 1-5.

Galvin, G. & Timmins, F. (2010). A phenomenological exploration of intellectual   disability: Nurse's experiences of managerial support. *Journal of Nursing Management, 18*(6), 726-735. doi:10.1111/j.1365-2834.2010.01101.

Gilmore, D. S. & Bose, J. (2005). Trends in postsecondary education: Participation within the vocational rehabilitation system. *Journal of Vocational Rehabilitation, 22*(1), 33-40.

Hewitt, P. (2010). Nurses' perceptions of the causes of medication errors: An integrative literature review. *MEDSURG Nursing 19,* 159-168.

Ijiri, L. & Kudzma, E.C. (2000). Supporting nursing students with learning disabilities: A metacognitive approach. *Journal of Professional Nursing, 16*(3), 149-157.

Kolanko, K. (2003). A collective case study of nursing students with learning disabilities. *Nursing Education Perspectives, 24*(5), 251-256.

McCleary-Jones V. (2008). Strategies to facilitate learning among nursing students with learning disabilities. *Nurse Educator, 33*(3), 105-106.

Sharpe, M. N., Johnson, D. R., Izzo, M., & Murray, A. (2005). An analysis of instructional accommodations and assistive technologies used by postsecondary graduates with disabilities. *Journal of Vocational Rehabilitation, 22*(1), 3-11.

Simons, M. (2010). A procedure for providing advice and support for nurses with a disability. *British Journal of Nursing, 19*, 712-715.

Unver, V., Tastan, S., & Akbayrak, N. (2012). Medication errors: Perspectives of newly graduated and experienced nurses. *International Journal of Nursing Practice, 18*, 317–324.

Suggested Reading

Cortiella, C., Horowitz, S.H. (2014) The State of Learning Disabilities: Facts, Trends and

Emerging Issues. New York: National Center for Learning Disabilities. Retrieved on March 8, 2014 at http://www.smcoe.k12.ca.us/spedtf/Documents/State%20of%20LD%20 FINAL%20FOR%20RELEASE.pdf

6 TRIUMPH IS '*UMPH*' ADDED TO 'TRY': NURSING WITH HEARING LOSS

By Eloise E. Schwarz, RN-BC, MBA, CCM

My upbringing was similar to other families during the 1950's—large families, hand-me-downs, Sunday church services, and meals with the family every day. There were the weekly piano lessons, playing made-up games outside when not studying or cleaning my room, seeking opportunities to watch a garden spider spin her web, or trying to catch a firefly at dusk. Life was simple then.

Dreams of what I *grow-up to be* were fashioned and shaped by circumstances and people who played prominent roles in my life. Broken bones, closed-head injuries and super infections also influenced the directions I would later take. Teachers, nurses, educators, and expectations found in my family structure, facilitated a nurturing and safe environment.

Job roles/responsibilities played heavy in how I learned and adapted to the world that was doing an about-face with technology that began with my transistor radio and ended up with the FM system of today, my PC, 3G smartphone, and digital programmable hearing aids.

Experiencing three motor vehicle accidents with varying levels of physical trauma interrupted my elementary and secondary education. High school became a nightmare. I managed as best as I could in fine arts and mathematics; subjects that didn't require lots of hearing or verbal interactions. My focus was to complete the assignment with every available resource at my disposal and try my best to make a higher grade in comparison to the last that I received. Repetition became my middle name—writing to perfection or even playing piano—often driving everyone nuts in our household.

To pay for gasoline for the car, or tuition for school, working was a must. My first job was in housekeeping at a nursing home. There, my eyes were opened beyond what I knew of the profession. My maternal grandmother was a nurse at the old St Mary's Hospital in Milwaukee so I was intrigued by what was offered in this noble profession.

There are no shortcuts to any place worth going

I managed nursing school as best as I could and continued working at various nursing homes in different capacities. I worked hard at everything… sometimes to exhaustion. Not truly understanding how hard it was just trying to hear everything and appreciate a classroom discussion, or a teacher who spoke softly or just trying to hear anything in its entirety in any daily activity, made me all the more passionate to succeed. But deep down, I was beginning to think there was definitely something wrong with me.

My thinking process took longer than others I knew. Chalking it up to post-brain injury affects, I was determined not to be out of the game, just because of a speed bump in my life. I would set goals for myself and do them—no matter what. Accommodations were made through my own actions, perseverance, and a steely determination.

Triumph is just 'UMPH' added to 'try'

I was married, raising a child, and going about the business of working as a registered nurse. I would show everyone that I could do anything just like everyone else, even though it took longer or was more difficult for me. I made it work for me for 15 years. Then burnout took over. A work injury in 1988 took me out of the clinical setting and into the business world of insurance. I was working for a large national insurance company as a certified case manager. There, my hearing loss was discovered.

Wow… I can't hear… on the telephone! My work depended entirely on use of the telephone. So it involved me communicating with others, taking a profuse amount of notes for everything and anything, just so that I could hear and understand what was needed to do my work. Our meetings were rough. In retrospect, I can now understand why I was frustrated, sad, overwhelmed and yet determined to learn as much as I could with whatever

I could muster. No one ever mentioned to me **ever** that I wasn't hearing everything. But in actuality I wasn't like others. I didn't like this at all. So much work and still being two or three steps behind, left me with self-doubt, fewer friends, and threats of being laid off or fired. Whispering peers were the enemy as were conversations that I could not fully hear.

My employer at that time paid for my first pair of hearing aids, which I later found out were not the correct ones for my level of hearing loss. Dealing with my new role as a nurse with a disability did little to help me hear in my world of work. No one was there to help me understand and work through the grieving process of my loss. I was left in the position of taking sides—either in the hearing world or the "disabled" non-hearing world. Suddenly, I was faced with a label I didn't want. It felt distasteful; I denied the hearing loss by hiding my aids; and I defiantly acted as if it was all a mistake. I continued to act as if it was never my fault and everyone else had the problem, not me.

My hearing loss is genetic from birth, with additional assault from the three head injuries, toxic side effects from high-dose antibiotics for sepsis treatment postsurgery, as well as from noise exposure. Once the hearing hair cells are damaged or blown away, they are gone forever.

I applied to a master's degree program and won entry to the master's in business administration (MBA) – Health Care Administration Program at Concordia University, WI. This would be my test to prove that I could do it, despite not hearing well.

Perseverance is not a long race - it is many short races – one after another

Even though I was experiencing rejection, alienation, abandonment, and a whole host of psychological and physical feelings, I would stay the course. After all, I was a nurse with a business degree. I could make things right. Unfortunately, the world didn't see it that way.

While we have legislative rules and regulations that speak on behalf of those who have disabilities, it doesn't always work well, easily or as intended in the workplace. While I knew that the laws were there, trying to understand and apply them in real life, didn't work for me.

Working full time while attending school full time and managing a household as well, made me a "super woman" who had a hearing impairment— and got by anyway. It was difficult but I managed with lessons learned, enthusiasm, and the fortitude to do anything.

Daring to finish my master's degree in record time (three years) without accommodations is in itself remarkable. The university accommodated the deaf but not the hard of hearing students. If I had known that there were ways to help me, I would have asked. But unfortunately, the national awareness and proclamation for accommodations at the local level was years away. We are only now just starting to awaken the giant.

For my efforts, I earned the MBA Student of the Year award given by the university. I was incredulous that anyone cared or took notice but at the same time, I was honored.

Balancing between working with all the tricks I learned, and taking the route of resistance in asking for accommodations was both tedious and difficult. I did not know enough about hearing loss; and I did not take the time to really investigate it—both parts of denial. I knew I had a loss in both ears, the loss had been from birth, and that I would always need some type of hearing instrumentation.

How is it that as a nurse I could help others but not myself with my hearing loss? Was it beneath me to ask or inquire about how to take care of me? I really preferred doing things my way… on the edge of daring… but still following the expected rules. We all have options and choices that we don't always like or want to act on, but if we value the life that we are given, then why not tackle one more speed bump?

My faith, family, and close friends over the years have helped me to move forward. Nothing has been denied to me, except for a few jobs that were not meant for me anyway. Over the past 10 years, I have applied for any and every type of job possible for a nurse. I have experienced rejection, downsizing, upsizing, and firings over the last 30 years of my nursing career. Now I can understand why, in retrospect, those pent up frustrations and setbacks really were a part of the hearing-impaired experience. But my dreams to at least try and do anything helped to mold and answer the questions I pose every day to myself.

The only disability in life is a bad attitude

Alongside feeling distraught and put out because I was categorized as hard of hearing, I withdrew from others—my working peers, who I perceived as the enemy, and searched for new ways to learn, stretching my wherewithal into new worlds that I had never considered before. I became a guru of Internet research on hearing loss.

Since I was gaining a newfound skill of research, writing, and publishing (a children's book on nursing for my graduate school thesis; guest commentating for Medscape Nurses (Schwarz, 2003); promoting involvement at the legislative level; and quarterly insurance newsletters for members and providers), I could expand this capability. I was already writing weekly broadcasts for an online education website for case managers—why not widen my scope to include our state and federal legislators?

I began meeting legislators at town hall meetings and asked for accommodations (captioning) for their meetings with the public. They were more than happy to accommodate. I had the chance to collaborate with their staff and found what worked with the political scene. I made a name for myself. They understood my stand on issues that affected my life and indirectly, theirs.

I continue to write letters of support, encouragement, or dismay at the actions legislators are taking on my behalf (as well as for all of us). I was very happy to have the ADA amended in 2008 (but became effective in 2009). Congressman Jim Sensenbrenner (R-WI), one of the co-authors of the bill, knew me well from speaking to him of the difficulties I encountered. A framed letter of proclamation is hanging on my wall from President Bush and Rep. Sensenbrenner commemorating its passage.

Hearing aids and equipment are not considered medically necessary by the federal government (Medicare coverage). Despite research that shows what hearing instruments can do, coverage isn't available unless the state has legislation stating so. With Medicare setting the standards for coverage, hearing aids for the majority of the population in the United States is not a covered benefit. I continue to pursue the need for this legislation.

At the state level, I began working with my governor to consider a bill that would have all insurance companies cover hearing aids for children. After a long two-year battle for passage, the bill gained approval from both houses and the governor's signature in 2009. A major victory was won for our children.

Even with my hearing aids, I can't always hear well enough to interact with a room full of noisy people. I would much rather use my exuberance in my writing to identify lopsided decisions and rulings made by political leaders. It pays to speak up. Because of my efforts, I was appointed to the governor's Council for the Deaf and Hard of Hearing, as well as the Wauwatosa Citizens with Disabilities Committee.

As a nurse, I have always encouraged my patients to consider and join a support group. But I was reluctant. Finally, I joined a national/state and local support group for people who are hard of hearing. The Hearing Loss Association of America (HLAA) was a tool for my learning, growth in acceptance of my hearing loss and provided access to a new arena of people who shared the same limitations. With my enthusiasm and organizational skills, I became a voice in this organization. I sit on the HLAA Board of Trustees for the state and serve in a local chapter as well. I participate in activities that help spread the word about how to prevent hearing loss as well as how to work with those with hearing loss.

Flexible people never get bent out of shape

My clinical audiologist keeps an eye and ear out for my hearing needs: testing my hearing yearly via audiogram, etc.; assuring my hearing hasn't changed; and that my digital equipment is working appropriately. Being available to fine tune or correct the electronics when needed are considered standard requirements and help assure I am equipped to go about my business. With the digital behind-the-ear hearing aids, I can go about my work relatively easily. The aids have different channels for listening depending on the environment, and they can work with other assistive listening devices.

These hearing instruments are my third set of hearing aids because my hearing loss is getting progressively worse. Hearing aids are not meant to last forever. The technology changes and hearing loss may change over time. The need for other types of instrumentation may be needed down the road, i.e. cochlear implants (CI).

Only you can be yourself. No one else is qualified for the job.

Family members were incredulous when I was first diagnosed. Suddenly springing this on to them made it hard for them to believe. But time and "show and tell" about what I was experiencing has helped to make them better understand. But often those who are closest forget. In my experience, it was too easy for them to point fingers and make fun of misstatements or mispronunciations of words.

Friends have come and gone depending on where I work. Most of the time, my work life has little to do with my home life. Patients have offered me more support and encouragement than my peers.

As time went on, my capabilities were slowly slipping away as the hearing loss became more pronounced. Over the years, I have sustained ridicule, pity, disdain, and other cruel criticisms from classmates, peers, friends, and managers, who should have known better but were too easily pulled into the fray. Why not? "She can't hear anyway!" they would say.

It's my belief that my master's degree brought on an even more intense dissatisfaction from those I worked for and with. I had not yet armed myself with the ability to disallow the snide remarks. I found myself without a job four different times in five years.

My hearing loss comes with a short-term memory loss mainly due to the intense concentration it takes to hear and synthesize every word spoken.

My verbal response may or may not be correct depending on what I understand. My delay is five to nine seconds, which is normal for hearing impaired people. Any delay in giving my response is an apparent cause for concern from others, unless I am able to fill in the awkward silence.

I have found the best approach is informing those who are conversing that I have a hearing loss and providing them with simple steps to aid me. I watch people's faces and try to be as close as possible to the conversation. Validating what is said helps move the conversation along.

There are spaces between our fingers so that another person's fingers can fill them in

Hearing loss is nothing to be ashamed of or apologize for. Admitting to having a hearing loss can take time and courage. Information is growing every day. Deaf and hard of hearing issues are being researched and assessed continually at the National Institute on Deafness and Other Communication Disorders. Special interest groups, institutions, and foundations are championing the cause in bringing information to the forefront of America's consciousness.

Accommodations in nursing will continue to be challenging but with them— more and more nurses with hearing loss are able to practice in a variety of settings. Learning about your hearing capability and exploring the equipment and accessibility services that you need is the first step to take. Utilizing the resources that are available should help your learning and understanding of the challenge.

If you have or suspect a hearing loss, network with other nurses with hearing loss and learn about amplified stethoscopes and other aides for clinical practice. Learn from the experiences of others. Visit www.ExceptionalNurse.com and the www.amphl.org. The Job Accommodation Network provides information workplace accommodations: http://askjan.org/

Look to our historical heroes and heroines, who despite their limitations were still able to overcome and change history. This is not the time to sit back and let someone else do the work. Taking the first step is a giant leap and one that will change your world. This is the time to plant the seeds of hope. Exciting times are ahead.

Come join me in the walk of a lifetime.

Building Resilience

Feel like something isn't right? Get a complete physical

Consider a job coach

Extend a hand to other co-workers

Don't apologize for hearing loss

Inform others how to work best with you

Utilize all available resources

Join a support group

Find your niche

Build on your strengths

Avoid the blame game

Be part of the solution

Eloise Schwarz is past-president of the Hearing Loss Association –Wisconsin and a QI Delegation Coordinator at Independent Care Health Plan in Wisconsin. She can be reached at Eloise6376@wi.rr.com.

Suggested Reading

Carmen, R., (2004). *The consumer handbook on hearing loss & hearing aids – A bridge to healing.* Sedona, AZ: Auricle Ink Publishers.

Hearing Loss Association of America, Bethesda, MD, www.hearingloss.org

Kaplank, H., Bally, S., & Garretson, C. (2007). *Speechreading – A way to improve understanding.* Washington, D.C.: Clerc Books, Gallaudet University Press.

National Institute on Deafness and Other Communication Disorders, Resource Directory, U.S. Department of Health and Human Services, www.nidcd.nih.gov

Schwarz, E. (2003). The nursing shortage: A call to action. *Topics in Advanced Practice Nursing eJournal, 3*(2) Retrieved on July 17, 2013 at http://www.medscape.com/viewarticle/453336.

COMMENTARY

By Leslie Neal-Boylan, PhD, APRN

Eloise's experience echoes the experiences of many nurses with disabilities. Initially, Eloise had to adjust to the diagnosis of hearing loss: "I denied the hearing loss by hiding my aids; and I defiantly acted as if it was all a mistake," and then she had to find ways to compensate so that she could do everything she wanted or needed to do. Nurses with disabilities tend to try to hide them partly out of fear of not getting a job or retaining a job, and partly because they are reluctant to display weakness.

Like so many other nurses with physical and/or sensory disabilities, Eloise experienced "ridicule, pity, disdain, and other cruel criticisms." She admits to having withdrawn from her working peers because of her diagnosis and because she saw them as the enemy. Yet, also like so many other nurses with disabilities, she refused to ask for accommodations and thought she could "do it all." I coined the phrase "nurse heroics" to describe how nurses, in general, whether or not they have disabilities, seem to feel they must sacrifice their own well-being or they cannot be good nurses.

This is particularly true of nurses with disabilities because they are reluctant to ask for accommodations. Nurses feel guilty taking their coffee breaks or going to lunch even when these are opportunities given to every employee. "Following the expected rules" is something nurses do because we have a keen sense of responsibility that is admirable, but sometimes it clouds our judgment with regard to looking out for ourselves.

Many nurses with disabilities, such as Eloise, channel their feelings about having a disability into joining organizations or supporting legislative or policy changes. Some nurses go back to school and find that the master's degree enables them to remain in nursing regardless of their disability. While they may experience discrimination during their schooling, they often find satisfaction in the new role. However, sometimes a period of "proving oneself" is required. Nurses with disabilities should not have to prove themselves any more than those without disabilities. Yet, for some reason, people assume that a physical disability impairs one's intellect or expertise.

Eloise admits to being aware of "legislative rules and regulations that speak on behalf of those who are disabled.... While I knew that the laws were there, trying to understand and apply them in real life didn't work for me." It is not uncommon for nurses with disabilities to be unaware of the details of the Americans with Disabilities Act that apply to their situations or to take advantage of their disability rights or the Family Medical Leave Act. I have also learned thorough many interviews with nurses with disabilities that they rarely consult an attorney regarding how they have been treated or explore whether the organization is treating them fairly based on the law. I think this stems from the inherent nature of nurses not to cause problems but to solve them.

Eloise offers readers a glimpse into her struggle, burgeoning awareness, and eventual strength and success as a woman and a nurse with a disability. Her experience mirrors those of many other nurses with disabilities. However, her efforts to enact change for people with disabilities and her own personal and professional successes should inspire and encourage other nurses with disabilities who may think they cannot or should not remain in nursing. Her experience should also help illustrate to employers that nurses with disabilities are valuable contributors to the workplace and that every effort should be made to hire and retain them.

Leslie Neal-Boylan is the associate dean and professor, school of nursing, Quinnipiac University, Hamden, CT. She is the author of numerous publications related to nurses with disabilities and the book Nurses with disabilities: Professional issues and retention *(2012) New York: Springer. She can be reached at* <u>ljboylan@quinnipiac.edu</u>.

7 UNLIKELY GIFTS: NURSING WITH DIABETES

By Siana Wood, BA, RN

Since the summer of 1983, I wanted to care for patients. I was eight years old and vacationing with my family in Canada, hundreds of miles from our home in the United States. I planned to swim and play with my brother and Canadian cousins, gleefully expending the summertime energy I'd saved up over the school year.

But during the preceding spring, I began to feel tired all the time and developed an unquenchable thirst. By summer, I was severely ill, and needed medical treatment for what we'd soon learn was juvenile (insulin-dependent, type 1) diabetes. I was diagnosed and treated at McMaster University Medical Center in Hamilton, Ontario.

Although my family and I were suddenly thrust into the complex realm of a strange disease, with its web of medical terms and new concepts, we were fortunate to be guided by a remarkable clinician and healer named Angus MacMillan, MD. Dr. MacMillan's approach to my diagnosis, and my family's unique situation as visitors in another country, considered all the variables involved in making the experience as positive and unencumbered as possible. Bucking standard practice, he arranged for me to be treated as an outpatient, figuring I'd want to go home with my parents each night, rather than stay in a strange hospital.

As time passed, I came to understand how profoundly Dr. MacMillan's guidance influenced my beliefs about living with and handling an illness. His trust in my abilities helped me develop a sense of strength and capability, even with a disabling illness regarded by many people as a tragedy. Along with a fascination for how the body works (and malfunctions), I developed the conviction that a collaborative combination of counseling, problem-solving, and support can be instrumental in helping individuals and families cope successfully with illness and the burdens that accompany it. I wanted very much to give those gifts to others.

It took me a long time to find the courage to go to nursing school. I earned a BA in liberal arts and worked for years in healthcare before I even considered becoming a nurse. What mostly held me back was concern about whether my health could withstand the stress of an unpredictable schedule, and where I'd find the money to attend school, and supplement any lost income from reducing my work hours. For years after completing my first degree in 1996, I requested brochures from nursing schools, dreaming and wishing, but never fully believing I could do it.

My Inspiration

I think what finally tipped the scale for me was the work of the nurses in my life. My aunt, a nurse and one of my biggest supporters, had been the one to recognize that something was seriously wrong with my health in the summer of 1983, and it was only because of her, that my family had sought urgent medical care for me. We have been close ever since, and she always encouraged me to go back to school for nursing.

Then, when I began working in a hospital as a project manager, I had access to a wonderful nursing leadership team who eagerly supported my dreams, patiently answered questions about nursing, and encouraged me to pursue a nursing degree. My aunt's message, amplified by other nurses, started to sink in. I started taking prerequisite science courses, and found I was in my element. When the hospital announced a special program to sponsor employees attending nursing school, it seemed meant to be. And so, 20 years after my diagnosis, I began the path to a nursing degree.

I have type 1 diabetes, the more rare of the two main types. Both type 1 and type 2 diabetes are about shortages of insulin, a hormone made by the pancreas and necessary for life, as it helps the body convert glucose into energy. People with type 2 diabetes still make some insulin, but their bodies have difficulty using the insulin they make. Those with type 1 diabetes make no insulin at all, and must replace their insulin with injections or subcutaneous insulin delivery. For both types, the goal is to try to maintain blood glucose levels as close to a person without diabetes as possible, because levels that are too low or too high are harmful. Unfortunately, this is so much easier said than done.

The medical world feels that type 1 is a more severe disease because the body makes no insulin at all, and thus it is harder to control the blood glucose. I'd have to agree, having lived with diabetes for 26 years. Producing no insulin, coping with the special effects of female hormonal cycles on diabetes, and tending to the complications I developed have made it a harder journey. To maintain tight glycemic control, it's necessary to do multiple finger stick blood sugars every day, weigh and measure food, calculate insulin doses, factor in exercise, stress, and illness, and try to adjust to unexpected changes. This is easier to do with an insulin pump, but it's still not the ideal system that "mother nature" intended with a functioning pancreas.

Required Attentiveness

The constant vigilance required of people with diabetes becomes a never-ending conversation with yourself. The noise in my brain is always there as I calculate boluses, tweak basal rates, estimate carbohydrate counts, figure, analyze, and worry. On a day when I've done everything properly, I might delve into an informal root cause analysis of why my blood glucose might be off. Could I be ovulating? Was it the steroids in the inhaler that I only use every once in a while? Could I be digesting something extra slowly today? Maybe there was some additional sugar, syrup, or fruit juice in that meal I ordered?

The worry alone could be paralyzing, but because it's what I have to do to be healthy, I've learned to let a certain level of worry be part of my diabetes management, coexisting alongside a newer sense of self-advocacy that reminds me I'm doing the best I can.

As someone who strives for tight control of my diabetes, I still have normal fluctuations— the occasional low blood sugar or high blood sugar that needs correction. No one can predict or plan every single variable in life that affects diabetes, but with close monitoring, you can be mostly prepared to respond appropriately. Both situations (lows and highs) kick my energy to the curb and leave me feeling a little disoriented and tired. Thankfully, because those situations are not my normal state, I feel well most of the time and recover relatively quickly (20 minutes for a "low," two hours for a "high") from those peripheries.

Secondary Conditions

Even with tight diabetes control, the cumulative effects of normal fluctuations in blood sugar over many years (26 in my case) take their toll on the body. I was diagnosed with diabetic retinopathy when I was 22, about 13 years after my diagnosis. It was caught so early and monitored so frequently thereafter that I was able to have eye surgery at age 26 that helped halt the progression of the retinopathy. I lost some nighttime visual acuity and some peripheral vision. As I write this, at age 34, my retinopathy remains "nonproliferative." At age 32, I had an episode of diabetic macular edema in one eye, underwent eye surgery, and have not since developed any new edema. I did lose some central visual acuity in that eye, but not enough to affect my driving or my nursing practice.

Kidney disease is always a concern with long-term diabetics. In nursing school, during a stressful semester, I had an episode of subclinical microalbuminuria, which didn't recur, and was considered transient and stress-related. My kidney function since then has been normal. Neuropathic and arthropathic changes have been the most prominent of my diabetic complications. People with diabetes are prone to multiple kinds of neuropathy; I have mild compression neuropathies (carpal tunnel syndrome and ulnar neuropathy), moderate meralgia paresthetica (numbness, pain, and tingling in both thighs), and mild-to-moderate diabetic gastroparesis – delayed gastric emptying caused by autonomic neuropathy.

Diabetes has affected my hand joints the most, with stenosing tenosynovitis ("trigger finger") in most fingers, and "diabetic stiff-hand syndrome" in one hand. Multiple surgeries have helped release compressed nerves and tendons in my hands and fingers, and at this point, I can still manage equipment, write, and type.

Because type 1 diabetes is an autoimmune disease, those of us with the disease are prone to develop other autoimmune conditions. A few years ago, I was diagnosed with Hashimoto's thyroiditis (hypothyroidism caused by autoimmune destruction of thyroid tissue), which, like diabetes, is treated with lifelong exogenous hormone replacement. My endocrinologist screens me routinely for signs of other autoimmune dysfunction.

Complicated Health, but Mine

It sounds like a lot. But it rarely feels that way to me anymore, especially since making it through nursing school. I still feel jarred when a physician or someone new to my situation remarks on how much medication I take, or how complicated my health is. Maybe I've become so used to absorbing each new detail as it comes that it hasn't felt like a big weight. Certainly, it's hard when something "flares"—or when more than one thing with my health is happening at once. It's frightening; terrifying sometimes. But it's what I have, so I find my way, just as I always have.

Once I finally made the decision to pursue my nursing degree, I was nervous about how I'd withstand the rigors of nursing school (the 10- and 11-credit clinical and theory courses that lay beyond the science prerequisites). Taking a three-credit prerequisite class twice a week felt manageable. But late night classes, evening and weekend clinicals, the amount of studying required—I knew these would challenge my ability to control my diabetes as I also kept working and tried to stay connected with friends and family.

The clinical portion of my nursing program consisted of four semesters, and before the first (Nursing 1), I contacted the disability coordinator at my campus. We talked about what I'd need in terms of accommodations (for me, that amounted to permission to test my blood sugar whenever I needed to, including during exams, and permission to have food with me at all times and to eat as needed, including during exams and clinicals). The disability coordinator prepared a document each semester that documented my needs, and was approved by the nursing faculty chair. I brought the letter with me everywhere, but after the first couple of times showing it to nursing professors to remind them that I needed to have my blood glucose meter, glucose, and snack with me, they were used to it and the letter mostly stayed in my book bag.

Every clinical instructor I worked with was understanding and flexible regarding my diabetes. It became apparent very quickly that the physical nature of bedside nursing drastically dropped my blood sugars, so I learned to run temporary, decreased basal rates on my insulin pump when I knew there was a transfer or a bed bath coming. Still, even then, I couldn't anticipate every situation that might cause hypoglycemia, and so sometimes even with my best efforts, I'd still get hypoglycemic. I always kept glucose and snacks with me, and it was never an issue for me to sit down and regroup. I think the hardest part of those frequent low blood sugars was (and still is) the pressure I put on myself: *I'm not being there for my patients; I shouldn't need to have someone else covering for me.*

I was lucky to have a nurse practitioner and board certified fellow in diabetes management as my clinical instructor for Nursing 2. A clinician, researcher, and teacher, she was known for being tough but funny, an ardent diabetes advocate, and someone who looked out for me as a student with diabetes, but also pushed me to do my best. She understood how the chaotic schedule of a clinical floor could create the high and low blood sugars I sometimes struggled with, offered suggestions for managing my condition while in clinical, and reminded me of my strengths and also of the places I could become better and stronger, as a future nurse, a student, and someone with diabetes.

Helping Others Understand

During one of my teacher's class lectures on diabetes, she had me talk about living with diabetes. I expressed that diabetes is a continuous balancing act between factors that are constantly shifting—stress, your body chemistry, insulin, food, exercise, illness. And that much of that balancing is invisible to the rest of the world, which can make it a hard disease to understand; I think diabetes' invisibility has helped foster the myth that you "just take a shot and that's it." But because of the constant vigilance diabetes requires, and the complications we can develop (I explained that my eyes, kidneys, and nervous system have been moderately affected), it can make for a heavier burden sometimes than people realize. I also said that having diabetes has made me more health-conscious and disciplined, and in that way was something of a gift.

My classmates asked some questions afterward. I think it helped me to feel like I communicated a bit about what it feels like to live with this illness to peers that will undoubtedly, as nurses, take care of people with diabetes in their careers. It also helped me feel like I was seen a bit more clearly by them, something I don't know that I needed until I stood up to speak.

The times I chose to reveal my diabetes to patients on clinical rotations were usually related to those patients having diabetes themselves. In certain instances, it was appropriate to do some patient education about diabetes, and provide therapeutic conversation about the ups and downs of living with diabetes. One of my patients was a young woman in the intensive care unit. She also had type 1 diabetes, and had recently been pregnant. When she went into labor, she called for an ambulance and asked the driver to bring her to Women & Infants,' the local women's specialty hospital, because her pregnancy was high-risk, but the driver brought her to a closer community hospital. She had an emergency cesarean there, during which she sustained an undetected colon laceration. She went home and developed acute peritonitis, which is why she ended up in the ICU (of another local hospital). During the times she was lucid, she asked me about my insulin pump, and we talked about how her pregnancy and diabetes had affected one another. She seemed comforted to be able to talk about it with someone who could sympathize.

Sometimes, because of my own experiences with diabetes, what I was able to provide (beyond my student-nurse training) was a way to help my patient become his or her own advocate. People with chronic illnesses learn their bodies so well and often have a sense when something isn't right. I encouraged patients to listen to their bodies and trust their instincts, talk to their doctors, and not be afraid to ask questions if they weren't satisfied, or remained uncertain about their situation.

An Unexpected Gift

I think what I most often brought to my student nursing—and what I try to bring to my patients now—is my undivided attention and a willingness to listen to patients talk about being sick, being hospitalized, being frightened and powerless, and vulnerable. Whether illness comes in a chronic form or an acute form, it can turn your reality and security upside down. Tending to the feelings unleashed by illness is an important a part of my nursing care—as much as the medical and technical aspects of nursing. It's one of diabetes' gifts, I guess. I wouldn't have learned how crucial that therapeutic presence is unless I hadn't been such a grateful recipient of it from the beginning, and throughout my years as a patient.

The routine of nursing school, family, work, and diabetes had become so "normal" in its own way that once I finished nursing school and passed my boards, it took me a little while to realize that I was really, truly a registered nurse. In Rhode Island, you can search for RNs and other licensed professionals on the state's health department website, and in my first month or so as a new nurse, I visited there several times to look up my own name and see that it was real and official!

Getting a job as a nurse was not as easy as I'd hoped, however. Despite the "nursing shortage" that has persisted in our country, the economic downturn of 2008 and 2009 really affected job prospects for new graduate nurses. I graduated in December 2008 and passed my boards in February 2009. In that time, our little state saw hospitals begin to enact hiring freezes, postpone "new grad programs," and in general make do with less. Retired RNs came out of retirement to fill positions, and others who had planned to retire in 2009 decided not to. That meant the anticipated vacancies for new graduates were greatly reduced.

Finding the Right Position

I knew when I was searching for a job that I should likely avoid a medical-surgical nursing position since its pace had wreaked havoc on my diabetes control when I was in school. I loved the pace and nature of ICU, maternity, and perioperative nursing, however, and tried to search for positions in those areas, but they just weren't available. I initially accepted a position as a dialysis nurse in an outpatient clinic, but instead ended up taking a job at a subacute rehabilitation facility that paid more, offered better benefits, and came with a bonus.

Unfortunately, the pace and staffing ratios at the subacute rehab were worse than on a med-surg floor. The nurse-patient ratio was 1:16, and I immediately was concerned that I wouldn't be able to take adequate care of my patients and myself. Many patients were post-op, some were post-stroke or post-MI, some were on chemotherapy, and others had tracheotomies and tubes. Nurses rarely stopped to eat or take breaks, and in general seemed miserable. And despite promises to the contrary, I was precepted by a licensed practical nurse. After one day on the floor, I decided that I wasn't willing to risk patient safety, my license, or my health, and told the director of nursing that I couldn't be a staff nurse.

My background in healthcare quality management appealed to the director of nursing, and she offered me an opportunity to train as a minimum data set (MDS) coordinator. Having no other options, I agreed, and began working in the MDS office. The staff was very kind, and trained me well. I learned pretty quickly to perform the in-depth medical record searching that was required to complete Medicare assessments. However, it remained a concern among the staff that as an inexperienced RN, I might not have the patient care experience they felt was important in doing the job well. Despite the scarcity of full-time staff nursing positions for new grads, I knew I needed to find some kind of clinical work, even if it was only part time.

The Best of Both

The road led to a wonderful compromise, as it turns out. I accepted a full-time weekday position as a quality management data abstractor at Women & Infants' Hospital in Providence, RI. On the weekends, I work as a pediatric home care nurse. As an abstractor, I apply clinical nursing knowledge to an opportunity for improvement, examining the medical data, interpreting the results, and making recommendations for improvement. Because my nursing knowledge is still so new, I ask a lot of questions, read as much related clinical material as I can, and "absorb and observe" —the active watching and listening that I do as a newcomer to learn from the nurses and providers caring for our patients. My clinical experiences as a home care nurse help add to that expanding nursing knowledge, too. For now, it's a good balance that allows me to do meaningful nursing work in two different settings, while also optimizing my diabetes management.

I still yearn to work more frequently with patients, but I do think things happen for a reason. One of the biggest gifts I never saw coming is the realization that with a low-physical-impact nursing job, I can safely plan for having a baby—and know that if I do become pregnant, I work in an ideal environment for managing a high-risk pregnancy.

There is something spare and simple and life affirming about finding the ability to treasure even the smallest of gifts when things are hard. It is part of how I keep going, too, when my health gets difficult—or when life in general is difficult.

For a long time I wrote and performed poetry, and I'm as drawn to words, I think, as I am drawn to tend people who are ill and hurting. One of my favorite quotes (author unknown) is, "The willow knows what the storm does not: that the power to endure harm outlives the power to inflict it." Life inflicts all manner of harm—disability included—but in the face of the worst of it, I can still bend, still endure. Somewhere along the way, I realized that for me, my diabetes, with its challenges and unlikely gifts, is both the willow and the storm. I don't have to like what the storm wreaks—the pain, the limitations, the uncertainty—but I know there will be calm again—and beyond the calm, so much more.

Building Resilience

Consider alternative career paths

Compromise

Work with the disability services office and faculty

Share your challenges with others

Balance

Bend

Siana Wood, RN, lives in Rhode Island with her husband Mike and their four cats. She has worked as both a nurse abstractor and a home care nurse. Siana now works as a nurse case manager for a Patient Centered Medical Home, a primary care practice in RI. She can be reached at sianawood@cox.net.

COMMENTARY

By Linda Carter Batiste, JD

This chapter shows what a difference a supportive employment environment can make and how much initiative employees with disabilities often have to take to be successfully employed. The Job Accommodation Network (JAN), a free consulting service funded by the U.S. Department of Labor's Office of Disability Employment Policy, may be helpful in situations like this. JAN can advise about rights and responsibilities under the Americans with Disabilities Act (ADA), accommodation options, and how to request accommodations.

When dealing with conditions like diabetes that require some flexibility and stress avoidance, it's critical to find the right employer. Although the ADA requires employers to consider flexible schedules and use of leave time in some jobs, like nursing, employers often have valid business reasons to deny such accommodations. It's much easier if the employer already sees the value of workplace flexibility and has built it into workplace policies and culture. Siana seemed to recognize this and she sought out jobs and workplaces that enabled her to have the flexibility she needs.

Another thing this chapter brought up was dealing with stress. One of the things we always emphasis with our callers is that stress is subjective so when you need to avoid or minimize stress, you need to be clear with the employer what exactly is the source of the stress. Individuals sometimes think the employer should know the source without being told, but they usually do not.

Siana's discussion about disclosing to classmates and openly discussing diabetes with them was very interesting. This can sometimes be useful in the work environment too, but the employee has to initiate it because of the employer's ADA confidentiality requirements. Disclosure to coworkers can take place informally with individual coworkers or formally in an employer-sanctioned presentation. Disclosure is generally a personal decision that each person makes. JAN provides information regarding the pros and cons on how to disclose as well as some practical tips.

For more information, see "Dos and Don'ts of Disclosure" at http://AskJAN.org/media/disclosurefact.doc.

Siana also had good insight into what she needed in a work environment and what should be avoided. Sometimes individuals end up in exactly the wrong job and work environment with negative consequences to their health. She also took it upon herself to balance her work with her home life. This is usually the individual's responsibility and not something employers have to consider.

Linda Carter Batiste, JD, is a principal consultant with the Job Accommodation Network (JAN), a free consulting service funded by the U.S. Department of Labor's Office of Disability Employment Policy. She has in-depth training on the Americans with Disabilities Act (ADA) and employment law as well as accommodations related to mobility impairments, emergency evacuation, and substance abuse.

Suggested Reading

For information about accommodating employees with diabetes, see http://askjan.org/media/diab.htm

8 SICK AND TIRED OF BEING SICK AND TIRED: NURSING WITH LUPUS

By Pamela Delis, RN, BSN, MSN

Being a nurse with lupus can be a blessing. Why? Because you know what it is like to be sick and tired of being sick and tired. You know what it is like to have chronic joint pain, overwhelming fatigue, occasional cognitive lapses, and regularly scheduled laboratory tests. You have probably had people question your pain or illness because you don't look sick. You have experienced both the nurse and the patient role in the nurse-patient relationship. In other words, because of lupus you possess a better appreciation for what it is like to travel through the lonely, frightening, overwhelming roads of our healthcare system. It is said that what doesn't kill you, will make you stronger. I agree.

Lupus and (Perceived) Luck

First of all, let me say that I had reservations about telling my story. I don't consider myself having a disability. I read stories about the challenges that other nurses successfully rise above and I believe my situation pales in comparison. I consider myself fortunate; I have the support of my family and friends. I have the ability to follow my dream of graduate education. Lupus has taught me to take better care of myself because I have to. It has taught me to stay out of the sun, get the sleep I need, exercise, eat healthy foods, and to be a more compassionate, empathetic nurse.

I have lived my entire life on the North Shore of Massachusetts. I grew up in a lower middle class family that embraced a strong work ethic and personal responsibility. I worked through my high school years as a nursing assistant in a local nursing home to save money to put myself through college. The work was physically and emotionally taxing but I thoroughly enjoyed it. At the time, I vowed that I *"would never become a nurse,"* although I will concede that I also thought that if I did become a nurse I wanted to be like the two registered nurses who worked the evening shift. They were intelligent, kind, fun, and caring, and never hesitated to lend a hand to the nursing assistants. There was always a sense of "we are in this together" when they were on duty. I have tried to emulate this sense throughout my professional career.

My college life began at the University of Lowell in Massachusetts as a physical therapy (PT) major. Little by little, I began questioning my decision—something about PT didn't feel right to me. I not only desired to help others but the restless side of me desired a career that offered many challenges and opportunities. After much soul searching, I realized that I really did want to be a nurse after all. I transferred into the BSN program, graduated in 1982, and have been a nurse ever since.

My own road with systemic lupus erythematosus began many years ago. I worked my way through the ranks in long-term care nursing to a position as an assistant director of nursing. I worked at a local skilled nursing facility; it suited both my professional aspirations and my personal needs to work locally because I was mom to a preschooler. My husband was in the throes of a career change and was attending college, and subsequently attended law school. Money was tight but we were happy. My health was an issue, however. After struggling many years with endometriosis, I made the very tough decision to undergo a total hysterectomy.

In March of 1997, I had an abdominal hysterectomy with bilateral salpingo-oophorectomy. I expected a six-week recuperation period and then planned to continue with my full-time job as assistant director of nursing. My road to recovery wasn't that easy, however. Six weeks turned into months. I experienced overwhelming fatigue, anorexia with significant weight loss, strange rashes, joint pains that seemed to vacillate between mildly annoying to crippling, and cognitive problems with memory issues and word-finding problems. During the recuperative period, I also experienced a case of vertigo and developed interstitial cystitis.

A Tough Time

I felt like my world was caving in around me. I literally dragged myself into work where I couldn't stay awake past lunchtime. The director of nursing, the administrator and coworkers constantly expressed concern over my condition. The DON brought me a muffin to work every day because I was losing so much weight. A staff nurse brought me some crutches because I had terrible tendonitis in one of my hips. I had to officially drop my hours to 20 a week and I lost my ADON position. It hurt financially as well as psychologically. The worst part of this experience was in not knowing what was wrong with me.

I had physicians literally telling me that my problems were psychological, and questioning my reports of pain. More than one healthcare provider told me that all my symptoms were related to depression and that I needed counseling. I tried to tell them that I was depressed solely because I was so tired; I was not tired because I was depressed. My life revolved around work, my family, and many hours of sleep. I was so fortunate to have a husband, parents, and siblings who expressed concern and love throughout this period of my life. I was also lucky that I had a child who loved drawing, playing Legos, sharing books, and making puzzles; these were all things that were not physically taxing yet were fun and enjoyable for us both.

After what seemed to be an eternity, because of all my postoperative problems, my reproductive endocrinologist stated he thought that I had some underlying issue, perhaps of an autoimmune nature. My primary physician referred me to a rheumatologist who initially believed that I had fibromyalgia or some type of a connective tissue disorder. (My actual diagnosis of SLE didn't come for a couple of years.) He eventually started me on Plaquenil and approximately six months later, I actually started to feel better!

I slowly increased my hours back up at work and eventually became the director of nursing at the same facility. The administrator and the wonderful staff knew of my challenges and tolerated my lupus flares. I think my staff watched out for me as much as I watched out for them. The fact remained, however, that I was having a great amount of difficulty managing working the demanding hours, the stress that comes from worrying 24/7 about my residents and staff, and being a mom and wife. With very mixed emotions, I left my position for a district position in long-term care utilization and reimbursement. Unfortunately, even though this job didn't have 24/7 responsibilities, it did involve constant travel that I subsequently learned took its toll on my health.

Back to the DON

A year later, my old company wooed me back with an offer to become the director of nursing at another local facility that they had just acquired; I agreed to become the DON on a temporary basis. My six-month agreement lasted a couple of years! The reason I lasted as long as I did in this 24/7 role again was because of the support of the executive director and the nursing management team. As in my last DON position, the staff and I really took care of each other.

Unfortunately though, my body gave me a frightening wake-up call. My fatigue level had been climbing and while at work, I developed terrible chest pain. With my executive director by my side, I landed in the local emergency department and was diagnosed with pericarditis. My terrified son looked at me lying on the stretcher and asked "Mom, are you going to die?" Right then, I knew that I needed to find a better answer.

After recuperation, I stayed on with the company working reduced hours, doing a number of temporary positions mostly in performance improvement and reimbursement. There was no job security with these temporary positions, and although I excelled at leadership level positions in long-term care, the truth was that I found the hours and traveling to be too much of a challenge for me.

I left long-term care and took a position working for the executive director who had been by my side in the emergency room. She had left long-term care and was working for the local hospital. Part of the hospital's plan was to develop a Medicare-certified home health care department. I was brought in on a management level; although the position was full time, I believed that working locally again with little 24/7 responsibility would be a good fit for me. I enjoyed the new challenge of applying my skills in a new arena. My boss and I continued to have a great working relationship.

All was going fine until I fell in the snow and shattered my distal radius of my left arm. I required surgery with plates and screws. Again, as before, my recuperation took much longer than I had hoped for, and I ended up in months of occupational therapy. I worked part-time, went to therapy, napped, and cared for my family.

Turning Lemons into Lemonade

Unfortunately during this time, my position was cut due to budget issues. I was distraught. For the first time in my life, I was unemployed! I was still recuperating, trying to find a job that was a good fit for my talents and my health needs. It was a period of angst that led me to make a decision that brought me forward to a lifelong dream.

I decided to take on the challenge of returning to acute care. I enrolled in and successfully completed a clinical refresher course and subsequently returned to acute care nursing on a part- time basis. Although I certainly revealed my diagnosis on my pre-employment health questionnaire, I have purposely kept my diagnosis of lupus from my coworkers. I often feel guilty that I do not volunteer to stay extra shifts or pitch in with the 11-7 call-ins; although I know that I need to watch out for my health. While I am at work, I give 100 % to my patients and my coworkers.

What I have found is that we all have challenges we bring to work with us; sometimes they are the challenges of a chronic illness, and sometimes they are the challenges of everyday life. To be successful as a unit, we must capitalize on each other's strengths. Although I am not the strongest, physically, nor have the most stamina, I excel at working with patients and families that others may find challenging. I am great at listening and problem solving and often find that even the most demanding patients just want someone to take their concerns seriously. I have great empathy for those in pain, and because of my years in gerontology, I also have empathy for the elderly and chronically infirmed.

One patient I will not forget was a woman who was in her seventies. I had been told in report that she complained of a lot of fatigue. I looked at her diagnosis list and had a pretty good idea I knew why. When I went into her room that afternoon, she was sitting up in the chair next to her bed with her eyes closed. I went in and introduced myself as her evening nurse. I checked her IV, took her vital signs, completed her assessment and then sat down next to her and asked about her fatigue. She said that no one understood how tired she was.

She described the fatigue as "hitting the wall." She said that it was hard to keep her eyes open after lunch. She said she realized the need to stay out of bed and to walk around, but she was so tired she found it quite difficult. I asked her if she thought it was because of her lupus and she said that she was quite sure it was. She talked about periods of feeling well, and then periods of overwhelming fatigue. Then I did what I had never done before; I told my patient that I, too, had lupus. I told her that I, too, had experienced the overwhelming kind of fatigue that she described and I understood what she meant by "hitting the wall." I remember her regarding me with a look of awe and saying "You have lupus and you're a nurse? You really do understand!"

We developed a fond rapport, and each day her fatigue abated. I had made sure that I passed on in report her need to alternate periods of activity with periods of rest because of her lupus. She recuperated slowly but surely and was subsequently discharged home. I knew that I had pushed the boundary of the nurse-patient relationship by revealing my own diagnosis of lupus, but my instinct told me that it was the correct thing to do in this particular situation—this patient who felt so alone in her battle with fatigue.

On to Graduate School

During this time in 2007, which was 25 years after graduating from college, I finally went back to school for my master's in nursing science degree. Graduate school has been a dream of mine for many, many years. Family, health, and financial constraints had always stood in my way. But my son was finishing up his high school years, my husband had a successful business and I was fortunate enough to be able to focus on my own career aspirations. Graduate school was definitely rigorous but I met such a dedicated group of nurses with such a diversity of skills and strengths, it was uplifting. Now I'm furthering my education in a PhD nursing program.

Balancing family, school, and work challenges excites me. I aspire to teach students with all sorts of strengths and challenges, and to groom them to become the kind of intelligent, caring, and empathetic nurses that our patients deserve.

Advice to Nurses

What message would I like to offer other nurses and students with their own health challenges? Be patient with yourself. Persevere. Try to focus on all the things you CAN do, all of your strengths. Don't be afraid to try new things; there are so many avenues in nursing. Read nursing journals. They offer up-to-date clinical information and often have articles about types of nursing that you have never considered before. If possible, continue your education. A higher education offers so many more career options. There are many online educational opportunities that exist for nurses. At the very least, keep your skills current with continuing education. Join professional nursing organizations and advocate for change.

Be creative in both your career and in your daily practice. Nurses excel at creativity and at "making do" with what we have. We teach our patients how to get out of bed after a cerebral vascular accident; we educate patients with vision impairment how to manage insulin injections. We need to tap into our inner reserves to hold our heads high and see our own worth.

What I have found through the many years of trying to find the right fit for my nursing abilities, is that the more I angst over career decisions, the less clearly I can envision the future. Too often I have focused on what I can't do instead of what I can. Our patients need nurses like us who have experienced firsthand what it is like to navigate through our lonely and often overwhelming healthcare system.

To the nursing profession as a whole I would say this: We need to support each other and break through barriers that impede the nurse with a disability from finding gainful, enriching employment, as well as what prevents the nursing student with a disability from successfully joining our profession. Too often, those with disabilities and work-related injuries are left behind. We need to advocate for accurate job descriptions; in my experience, they often list demanding physical requirements that are not truly necessary for successful completion of job duties. We need to begin to look at job requirements and find creative solutions that would enable more skilled, yet disabled, nurses to re-enter the workforce.

As a profession, we need to ensure that technology and equipment is available that will assist nurses with special needs to care for their patients. Let's face it: The average age of nurses in this country is continually climbing. There will be highly skilled nurses facing the physically demanding tasks that presently now pervade many avenues of nursing. We need to develop avenues for education that prize the strengths of nurses while affording less physically demanding opportunities.

On the state level, the Board of Registration in Nursing has a dedicated program to assist those nurses with substance abuse problems to get back into the workforce; this is a positive approach to a real problem. Is this a viable approach to assist those with a myriad of other health concerns? I don't know. I do know that creativity and innovation are key to keeping a diverse nursing workforce employed.

At the beginning of this story, I said that being a nurse with lupus can be a blessing. I am a better nurse because of my lupus. I understand the fear that comes from undiagnosed health problems, the anxiety of awaiting laboratory results, the frustration of not being taken seriously. I empathize with my patients who are tired of dealing with a chronic illness and the insecurities it brings. I believe my patients' reports of pain and I know that looks can deceive. I understand the need for control over one's experiences. I can appreciate the overwhelming, "hit the wall" kind of fatigue that some patients experience. And, I know the healing power of listening and presence.

Am I glad that I have lupus? No. Am I ever discouraged, sick of being sick and tired of being tired? Yes, definitely. But this is one of my life's challenges and I am sure that there will be many more. I am a nurse who happens to have lupus. I try to learn from my own experience of living with a chronic illness and I think that I am a better nurse because of it.

Building Resilience

Further your education

Morph your skills into another nursing specialty

Reinvent yourself

Focus on your strengths

Recognize that everyone has challenges

Pamela Delis, MSN, RN, is currently undertaking PhD in nursing studies with a focus on health promotion at the University of Massachusetts/Lowell. She is a full-time faculty member for the school of nursing at Salem State University, and works part time as an RN for children with developmental disabilities. She lives in Massachusetts with her husband, dog, and two cats. Her son is away at college pursuing pre-medical studies. She can be reached at pam@mac3.net.

The Exceptional Nurse

COMMENTARY

By Patricia K. Weinstein, PhD, ARNP, NP-C, CNE

Systemic lupus erythematous (SLE) is a chronic autoimmune disorder with estimates of prevalence rates in the United States ranging from 15 to 103 per 100,000 persons. (Ward, 2004; Furst, Clarke, Fernandes, Bancroft, Greth, & Iorga, 2013). No statistics exist on the prevalence of SLE among nurses, but it is possible to extrapolate an estimate using data from the Nurses' Health Study, which enrolled 184,643 female nurses without SLE at baseline between 1976 and 2004 and followed them for 11-21 years (Costenbader, Kang, & Karlson, 2010). Among that population, 192 women developed SLE with a resulting prevalence of 104/100,000. This number slightly surpasses the current most generous estimates of physician-diagnosed SLE prevalence in the United States. Thus, it is possible that nursing may be disproportionately affected by lupus compared to other professions.

Most individuals with SLE are diagnosed between the ages of 15 and 40 (Petri, 2002). For many nurses with SLE, this is the same time that they are entering a profession they have spent years dreaming of and preparing for. SLE is a chronic, relapsing disorder with unpredictable manifestations that often vary within the same patient as well as from patient to patient. The uncertainty and relapsing nature of SLE makes it difficult for affected individuals to anticipate if and when they can fulfill professional responsibilities. Loss of job portends not only loss of income but also threats to self-image and loss of health insurance.

Patients with SLE often do not look ill. Despite high doses of steroids, some patients do not exhibit cushingoid features because of glucocorticoid resistance (Melo, Melo, Saramago, Demartino, Souza, & Longui, 2013). The malar rash characterized by a butterfly pattern of erythema over the cheeks and nasal bridge can be fleeting. Aching joints typically are not deformed. Renal involvement is not obvious until renal failure becomes an issue. Public knowledge about SLE is lacking, but sadly, even many nurses are not thoroughly informed. Most nursing programs devote only a few minutes to SLE when discussing autoimmune or rheumatologic disorders. Thus, complaints of fatigue, pain, and memory problems may be suspect by family, friends, and co-workers.

Pam's story of her lupus journey is not unusual—delayed diagnosis, fatigue, work challenges. Like many patients with SLE, Pam spent years trying to discover the source of her illness. There is no definitive diagnostic marker for SLE and the presenting symptoms are common to many disorders. The average time between initial presentation and definitive diagnosis is two years (Ozbek, Sert, Payda, & Soy, 2003). This is an improvement from 10 years ago when the average time to diagnosis was three to 10 years. For many, receiving the diagnosis of SLE provides relief— because it answers their questions.

Pam's approach to her disease—her creation of a new reality rather than succumbing to a path determined by her disease—is one I often have encountered among patients with SLE. Rather than dwelling on what has been lost, they seek different options, including professional ones.

According to the American Disabilities Act, some individuals with lupus will qualify as having a disability and others will not. The Job Accommodation Network (JAN) of the Office of Disability and Employment Policy of the U.S. Department of Labor provides information on assistive technologies and other accommodation options for individuals with disabilities and recommends that accommodations be made on a case-by-case basis that considers an employee's individual limitations and needs (Batiste, 2011).

Accommodations for SLE

Some options suggested for patients with SLE, such as providing access to a refrigerator, modifying the dress code and implementing ergonomic workstations can be implemented in many healthcare settings. However, others, such as installing low-wattage overhead lights, allowing longer breaks and flexible work hours, prioritizing job assignments, and use of a personal attendant may not be possible in a hospital setting. Therefore, whether a nurse with lupus will be able to continue to work depends upon his/her limitations as well as the workplace's capabilities to implement accommodations.

While nurses may be hesitant to disclose how they feel for fear of losing their jobs, Pam's story illustrates the benefits of working closely with your employer. Additionally, nurses should inform themselves of their rights under the Americans with Disabilities Act. Research has shown that SLE adversely affects careers, regardless of profession (Schneider, Gordon, Lerstrom, Govoni, Nikai, & Isenberg, 2011). Perhaps nurses are more fortunate than others in this respect since nursing offers many career paths outside of the hospital where jobs tend to be the most physically and mentally demanding. Less physically demanding positions include school nurse, office nurse or research nurse.

For those nurses who can return to work, it is essential to find a balance between work and taking care of oneself. This may entail not only seeking a nursing job that is less physically demanding or has fewer hours but also acknowledging the need for assistance and accepting offers of help—an often-difficult task for nurses who previously have been in control of their patients' healthcare. Some co-workers may resent what they see as special treatment, but nurses are generally known for their empathy and working as a team. Keeping supervisors and co-workers informed about changes in health status is necessary to maintain their support.

There is an expression, "Once a nurse, always a nurse." Nurses unable to return to work because of their SLE may grieve the loss of a profession and career they had worked so hard to attain and that is intimately intertwined with their self-image. This loss follows the grieving process and needs to be addressed. Professional counseling may be necessary (Antzcak, 1999).

Using Experience to Help Others

Perhaps a source of consolation is the fact that these nurses may still be able to use their nursing knowledge and expertise to help patients with SLE through their participation in lupus support groups, online support communities, and awareness activities sponsored by local, state, and national lupus foundations.

Pam writes of the importance of support from family and co-workers. Research supports a strong and consistent relationship between social support and disease activity, disease damage and quality of life in patients with SLE (Mazzoni & Cicognani, 2011). In order to provide support, family, friends, and co-workers need to know about SLE and its ramifications. Many organizations, such as the Lupus Foundation of America, provide educational materials for families of patients with SLE. Likewise, support groups welcome family member participation. Educational resources for nursing staff are available in various formats (see Suggested Reading).

Pam also describes the insight her illness has provided into the illnesses of her patients. As mentioned, nurses do pride themselves on their empathy for their patients but it is undeniable that shared experiences can heighten empathy. Pam's words are good advice for nurses who care for patients with SLE who may not necessarily look ill but nonetheless express complaints of fatigue, pain, and numerous other symptoms. Validation of symptoms alone can provide comfort.

The good news about SLE is that survival rates in patients in the U.S. have improved from 50% at 5 years in 1975, to 95% at 5 years and 78% at 20 years in 2004 (Doria, Zen, Canova, et al., 2010). In 2011, the FDA approved the first new drug for SLE in 50 years (Ledford, 2011), and several more are in the pipeline that promise disease remission with fewer side effects than steroids. The Department of Health and Human Services, Office of Minority Health has established the Eliminating Lupus Health Disparities Initiative, an initiative for increasing lupus education curricula among schools of medicine, nursing, allied health, and other practicing health professionals. The future holds hope for nurses with lupus.

Patricia K. Weinstein, PhD, ARNP, NP-C, CNE is a nurse practitioner and founder of a free lupus clinic for the uninsured at Shepherd's Hope Clinic in Longwood, FL. She is an adjunct faculty at the College of Nursing, University of Central Florida where she established the first liaison between a lupus foundation (Lupus Foundation of Florida) and a school of nursing (College of Nursing, University of Central Florida). This partnership supports lupus-related educational and research endeavors. Dr. Weinstein is also a board member of the Lupus Foundation of Florida, Education Chairman and Annual Seminar Coordinator. She has conducted research and authored many publications related to this topic. She can be reached at: Lupusnurse@gmail.com

References

Antzcak, M. (1999). Attending to the grief associated with involuntary job loss. *Journal of Pastoral Care, 53*(4), 447-60.

Batiste, L.C. (2011). *Job Accommodation Network. Accommodation and compliance series: Employees with lupus.* Retrieved on January 28, 2014 from http://askjan.org/media/lupus.html.

Costenbader, K.H., Kang, J.H., & Karlson, E.W. (2010). Antioxidant intake and risks of rheumatoid arthritis and systemic lupus erythematosus in women. *American Journal of Epidemiology, 172*(2), 205-16.

Doria, A., Zen, M., Canova, M. et al. (2010). Diagnosis and treatment; when early is early. *Autoimmunity Review, 10*(1), 55-60.

Furst, D.E., Clarke, A.E., Fernandes, A.W., Bancroft, T., Greth, W. & Iorga, S.R. (2013). Incidence and prevalence of adult systemic lupus erythematosus in a large US managed-care population. *Lupus, 22*(1), 99-105.

Ledford, H. (2011). First lupus drug in 50 years approved. *American Journal of Health-system Pharmacy, 68*(8), 646.

Mazzoni, D. & Cicognani, E. (2011). Social support and health in patients with systemic lupus erythematosus: a literature review. *Lupus, 20*(11), 1117-25.

Melo, A.K., Melo, M.R., Saramago, A.B., Demartino, G., Souza, B.D. & Longui, C.A. (2013). Genetics and Molecular Research, 013 Feb 19, 2012(AOP). (Epub ahead of print).

Ozbek, S., Sert, M., Payda, S. & Soy, M. (2003). Delay in the diagnosis of SLE: the importance of arthritis/arthralgia as the initial symptom. *Acta Medica Okayama, 57*(4), 187-90.

Petri, M. (2002). Epidemiology of systemic lupus erythematosus. *Best Practice & Research. Clinical Rheumatology, 16*(5), 847-58.

Schneider, M., Gordon, C., Lerstrom, K., Govoni, K., Nikai, M. &

Isenberg, D.A. (2011). The substantial negative impact of systemic lupus erythematosus on the working lives of patients: results of the Lupus European Online Survey. *Arthritis & Rheumatism, 63*, November, 2011 Abstract Supplement.

Ward, M.M. (2004). Prevalence of physician-diagnosed systemic lupus erythematosus in the United States: results from the third national health and nutrition examination survey. *Journal of Women's Health, 13*(6), 713-8.

Suggested Reading

American College of Rheumatology. http://www.rheumatology.org

Gorman, S. (2009). *Despite lupus: How to live well with a chronic illness.* ePublished: Four Legged Press.

Jackson-Ferguson, WM., Maheady, D. C. (April, 2006) Curb cuts. *Florida Advance for Nurses, 21-22.* Retrieved on January 28, 2014 from http://www.exceptionalnurse.com/pdf/except_nurse_curb_cuts.pdf

Job Accommodation Network. Accommodation and compliance series: Employees with lupus. http://askjan.org/media/lupus.html

Lupus Foundation of America. Information for patients, families and healthcare professionals. http://www.lupus.org

Department of Health and Human Services, National Institutes of Health, National Institute of Arthritis and Musculoskeletal and Skin Diseases. Lupus: A patient care guide for nurses and other health professionals, 3rd edition. http://www.lsnflorida.org/files/nurse_book-care_guide.pdf

Rheumatology Nurses Society. Professional and educational resources for rheumatology nurses. http://www.rnsnetwork.org

Rowshandel, J. (2012). Juggling job and lupus. *S.L.E. Lupus Foundation.* http://www.lupusny.org/about-lupus/coping-with-lupus-corner/juggling-job-and-lupus

St. Thomas Hospital, UK. Lupus: A guide for nurses. http://www.lupus-support.org.uk/Nurse/Nurse.htm

WebMD. Living with lupus (video). http://lupus.webmd.com/video/living-with-lupus

Wallace, D. J. (2008). *The lupus book: A guide for patients and their families.* New York: Oxford University Press.

9 NORMAL PEOPLE IN DIFFERENT WAYS: NURSING WITH MACULAR DEGENERATION

By Barbara J. Sainitzer, RN, BSN, MN

"Adapt, innovate and overcome"—how many times has my friend said those words to me when I found myself struggling to do something "the old way" instead of stopping and devising a "new way" to achieve whatever it is I want to accomplish? Since my progressive vision loss—I mean "loss of eyesight," not vision—I have had to learn the hard way: You can keep on doing the things you want to do; you just find new ways of doing them.

Although people with vision loss may not be able to "see" the details of a perfect sunset, they do have "vision" and can continue to serve and contribute to society. We just have to find new ways often with the help of others and resources like assistive technology.

I am a nurse who chose nursing because I sincerely wanted to help other people. I felt a calling. My parents, who were my role models, fostered that desire. The day when I received the letter of acceptance granting admission into my chosen hospital school of nursing was so exciting.

My early adult years might be considered pretty "normal." I graduated from nursing school, married, and started family life with three children.

During the time my children were growing up, I frequently inquired at the local university whether it was possible to register for part-time classes in order to earn my BSN degree. But the nursing curriculum required full-time classes at that time, so it seemed advancing to a BSN degree was always out of reach for me because I needed to work while going to school.

After my two oldest children graduated from high school, I learned about evening and weekend classes available at another university. At last, I had the opportunity to continue with gainful employment while taking classes towards an advanced degree.

Back in School

Initially, it was intimidating to enroll in college classes after being out of school for 25 years. However, I found it exhilarating and looked forward to each day. When my studies were completed for the BSN degree, I learned about a grant and stipend possibility for graduate school. Again, it was intimidating, but I took the Graduate Record Examination (GRE) and was admitted to graduate school the same year.

During the first few months of graduate school, my younger son was diagnosed with a terminal illness. In an effort to be strong for my son and the rest of the family, I sought help from my physician, who was very supportive. It was during that examination, she saw something that required an immediate consultation with an ophthalmologist. During the ophthalmologist appointment, I heard "…there is nothing that can be done and it is progressive…"

I could hardly believe what I was hearing when the ophthalmologist said, "You have macular degeneration. There is nothing that can be done about it. It is a progressive disease. I have a video in the next room for you to watch. The nurse will show you the way. I want to see you back in a year." Dutifully, I watched the video about macular degeneration with tears streaming down my face.

A Most Difficult Time

Here I was 48 years old, finally had a chance to pursue an advanced degree on a grant and a stipend; my 25-year old son was diagnosed with a terminal illness; and I was losing my vision.

Until that time, I had been blessed with 20/20 vision, and a loving family.

Admittedly, I bartered with God, "I know you aren't supposed to give us more burdens than we can bear but, give me a break, Lord. What am I to do?"

Many years have passed. My son did pass on within the year. My husband became ill. For about nine years, we dealt with Alzheimer's disease and all the complications until he passed on. I promised my son I would finish graduate school, which I did. I then relocated to a new community and began a new position at the age of 52.

The vision loss has been progressive over the years and has reached the point where I can no longer drive a car, read a book anywhere I choose, select greeting cards, or read labels on grocery store items but, I CAN read with the aid of assistive technology, use a computer and continue to be gainfully employed. The State Department of Services for the Blind has been a valuable resource.

Lessons Learned

I have learned to ask for help from others instead of being completely self-sufficient. I have learned that, when people KNOW that I have a visual impairment, most are more than willing to help. I have learned to take the bus. I have a cell phone with speech activation.

How did I learn what to do? I learned, by talking with other people and sharing resources.

One day while riding a bus, I started conversing with a woman passenger who was sightless and informed me of the local chapter of the American Council of the Blind. I am now on committees with the local chapter as well as the state chapter.

We are all unique individuals. My personal experience with visual loss has shown that often nurses are the least understanding regarding what a "disability" entails. Is it fear? Fear of not knowing how to talk with or just be comfortable around persons with disabilities?

All people experience hurtful remarks that can penetrate the inner core. One of the lessons to be learned from all of this is that we are all interdependent, and it can be a good thing to have to "ask" for help in order to give someone else the feeling of being useful and appreciated. Life is full of lessons, and we do need to keep "open" to others thoughts and feelings. Through awareness, we will learn that we are all "normal" people, just in different ways. The time to adapt, innovate, and overcome is NOW!

Building Resilience

Ask for help

Be part of the solution

Serve on committees

Communicate with lawmakers

Reach out to others

Advocate

Volunteer

Get Busy

Barbara Sainitzer was appointed in 2008 to the governor of the state of Washington's Committee on Disability Issues and Employment. Along with that position, she volunteers for the Washington Council of the Blind and serves on the environmental access committee. She also volunteers for the local chapter of the Council of the Blind and serves on committees at her church. She can be reached at SainB3@centurylink.net.

COMMENTARY

By Detra Bannister, RN

I was very sorry to hear about the traumatic loss of Barbara's son, husband and sight all wrapped into one long lasting event. People are amazing when they respond to such keen mental suffering the way she did. The triumphant outcome of keeping a promise and advancing her degree is tremendously healing and satisfying.

If you are now among the more than 25 million people in the United States living with vision loss, you need to know how important it is to find ways to accomplish routine tasks and goals. These are the skills that will enable you to live independently and productively, read and write, maintain a career—or launch a new one—raise a family, have a social life, travel, enjoy recreational sports, and games. In short, lead a normal life.

Go back and read Barbara's story. Get in touch with American Foundation for the Blind (AFB) CareerConnect mentors who, in spite of being blind or visually impaired, are working as nurses. They have already traveled this road. Volunteers in this program can help the nurse or nursing student who is/has lost sight sort through the twists and turns of navigating their way to a career in nursing (or back into one).

Questions to ask yourself: Do you want to stay in this field of nursing or use this as an opportunity to broaden your experience? Do you want to stay in nursing at all or use your skills to re-career? Be encouraged that accepting the fact that you may have to modify what you do in nursing or switch areas altogether is a winning strategy and not a defeat.

For example, after I lost my sight, I could not have continued to safely work as a scrub or circulating nurse in the OR, no matter what. However, I could transfer my nursing skills to other areas of nursing such as community or school health, which I did. Other people have chosen to open up a staffing business where they could still stay in touch with patients and those in need by providing them with competent nurses to fill a staffing need. Some people go into teaching, senior day care, legal nurse consulting, patient education or advocacy, etc.

Challenge Your Thinking

Be creative! Bend your thinking and get outside the box. Most of all, don't allow yourself to think for one moment that you cannot live independently and productively.

To employers, I would discuss strategies to incorporate nurses with disabilities into their workplace. Accommodations are typically inexpensive and easy to implement. They can be as simple as changing the lighting, trading job tasks with a co-worker, using a talking thermometer or lighted hand-held magnifier —they are not always expensive or complex.

If it turns out that the necessary accommodations are more expensive or high tech than the aforementioned ones, I would encourage the employer by sharing information like employers who hire disabled individuals are eligible for a tax credit in their business; and that, according to labor market studies, people who are blind or visually impaired (BVI) are more loyal employees as a whole than workers without disabilities. Also, based on a number of studies, workers who have a visual impairment have shown attributes that include a lower turnover rate and are on the high positive side of safe performance, productivity, reliability, and attendance.

Detra Bannister, RN has worked as a surgical, community and school health nurse. She works as a CareerConnect Program Specialist for the American Foundation for the Blind. She can be reached at careerconnect@afb.net.

Suggested Reading

AFB CareerConnect
Career Education and Exploration for People with Vision Loss
www.afb.org/careerconnect.org

AccessWorld
Technology and People Who Are Blind or Visually Impaired
www.afb.org/aw

The American Foundation for the Blind www.AFB.org

The Job Accommodations Network
(JAN)A service of the Office of Disability Employment Policy
www.askjan.org
Please also see chapter 14 written by Susan Nordemo, RN.

10 IF YOU CAN'T MOVE TO AUSTRALIA, FIND A GROUP OF AUSTRALIANS: NURSING WITH REFLEX SYMPATHETIC DYSTROPHY

By Lisa Lobdell, RN, BSN, MSN

Born in Newport Beach, California, I spent most of my life growing up in sunny, Orange County, in a warm, loving household with my parents, a younger brother, and sister. I am a 42-year-old nurse, who is energetic, adventurous, and a true optimist.

When I was 14 years old, I signed up at Hoag Hospital to become a candy striper. I put on the uniform with pride and zipped around the hospital taking specimens to the lab, transporting patients, and working in pediatrics. This experience was followed by a job working with patients with Alzheimer's disease at an adult day care center.

After graduating high school in 1989, I began preparing to become a nurse. Not just any nurse, mind you! I had high hopes of becoming the next Florence Nightingale. The journey started at a local community college, where I took all of my general education and prerequisite courses. School never came easy for me but through determination, tutors, and long hours of studying, I got through the classes and, in 1992, I started nursing school.

Little did I know the hard work was just beginning. I was absolutely terrified walking into a hospital and into a patient's room. When I was standing in front of my instructor, ready to give my very first injection, I looked like a deer in the headlights. I will never forget my patient's response when I asked her if the injection hurt. She politely reminded me that she was paraplegic and had no feeling. Oh….If I had a nickel for all the stupid things I said!

Military Nursing

In December 1995, I graduated with a bachelor's of science in nursing from California State University, Long Beach. About a year before graduation, a recruiter visited our nursing program. After her visit, it inspired me to join the military. I came home and called my friends and family to tell them the news. What an adventure it would be!! I soon visited Nellis Air Force Base in Las Vegas. I was taken to the Officers' Club where I felt I was stepping into the filming of "Top Gun." I did not need any further coaxing. I signed without reading all of the fine print.

On April 6, 1996, off I went joyful that I would meet my own Tom Cruise. I spent three years on active duty, and my rank prior to leaving the US Air Force was 1st Lieutenant, for which I feel honored, proud, and grateful. The things that I loved about the military are the many close friendships, the leadership skills I developed, and confidence gained in my nursing skills.

My ultimate goal was to travel, so I left the military and found a position as a nurse at Club Med followed by other positions as a traveling nurse. My travel assignments included: Hawaii, England, New York, and Australia. Each assignment brought new life experiences and adventures.

In Hawaii, I learned to make sushi and tried surfing. In England, I was able to travel around Europe. Back in the United States, I began an assignment in Manhattan about six weeks prior to 911 and worked and witnessed the tragedy firsthand. On arrival in Australia— I truly felt that I was home. I got to see my first kangaroo and koala in the wild and experience the fantastic beaches and people. Everything felt right. I loved my job and my boss. She worked with the staff to make sure we had plenty of time off. It seemed to be the perfect work/life balance.

My visa was only for a year stay, so when the time came, I felt the need to return home to family and friends. On my return to California, I took a position as a team leader for a medical group. I worked in a clinic with primary care, internal medicine, and pediatrics. After being home for several months, I decided I still longed to be back in Australia, so I decided to apply for permanent residency and return to my former job in Manly

Beach in Sydney.

Before starting my new life in Sydney, I planned to spend six months traveling the world. I went on safari for two months, came face to face with lions, and was escorted off a train in the middle of the night in Turkey due to a train crash.

But it was a step out of a small tour boat in Malaysia—that changed my life.

I missed one little step on the boat— fell— and heard a sound I never want to hear again.

Immediately, I knew it was serious. My friend hailed a cab and I was taken to the nearest emergency room. I was diagnosed with a bone chip fracture and put in a cast. This was my first fracture and it hurt, but we decided to continue our adventures and move on to Thailand.

A month later, I went to a hospital in Bangkok, Thailand, and had more x-rays taken. The bone chip was healing, and a walking cast was made. I was now able to bear weight as tolerated. After several weeks, I was still having a significant amount of pain. On return to Australia, I saw a family practice doctor, had more x-rays and then was referred to an orthopedic doctor…"stat." He told me I had a suspected avulsion fracture involving the Lisfranc ligament leading to joint diastasis between the first and second metatarsal with subluxation (dislocation).

A Shocking Discovery

It felt like time stood still when I heard him order an immediate CT scan and said probable surgery with at least three months off my foot. I almost fainted. As a nurse, I was used to hearing people receive bad news but was not used to being on the receiving end. My head spun, I felt like I was drunk and not in my own head or body.

Later, I found that the Lisfranc injury is named for the French surgeon Jacques Lisfranc in Napoleon's army. The injury is a fracture and dislocation of the joint between the forefoot and midfoot. The original injury described by Lisfranc usually occurred when a soldier fell from his horse, but his foot did not release from the stirrup. Today, the most common mechanism of this injury is when someone steps into a small hole, and the foot is unusually twisted with a great amount of force while pushing down. However, there are many other ways to sustain this type of injury (Cluett, 2013). It is a very serious fracture that requires immediate attention to prevent long-term complications.

I was set up for surgery in Australia and after six weeks of recovery, the surgeon cut the cast and I was able to fly back to California to finish convalescing. My plan was to return to Australia to begin work back in Sydney after my foot was healed. I began to appreciate the simple pleasures like taking a bath again… I realized all the things that I had taken for granted being a young able-bodied person. I had to use crutches for another four weeks. My parents bought me a wheelchair at a thrift store so that I could get out. The novelty of being on crutches had long worn out. As I started walking, I felt like a child learning to take his or her first steps. The fear of putting those crutches down and falling again was so real.

A Final Diagnosis

My recovery was further complicated when my foot would discolor as I put it on the ground, and the pain with walking was still severe. This situation led me to the veterans' hospital in Long Beach where the orthopedic doctor made a swift diagnosis of Reflex Sympathetic Dystrophy (RSD). These were three letters that I never wanted to hear. I had worked in trauma and knew how bad RSD could be.

I came home and had a good cry with my dog. Then, began the painful process of rehabilitation: physical therapy, occupational therapy, acupuncture, nerve blocks, medications, and every other kind of therapy that you can imagine. I began seeing one specialist after the next trying to find a way to help manage my severe, intense burning nerve pain.

My old boss called me up and said she put in a good word for me at the medical group. By the time I went back to work, it had almost been a year. They had an open case management position. I was lucky enough to be interviewed by a wonderful woman. As I walked with my cane, I felt less than adequate. I will never forget her for taking a chance on hiring me.

When I told her that I was having therapy, she told me that she could work with that. I felt fortunate, as I know that not all supervisors are willing to take on an employee with special needs.

Many times, I felt like I needed to overcompensate to prove that I could do it and to pave the way for other nurses with disabilities. I never called in sick. Pain was going to be a part of my life and I needed to deal with it. It would not be an excuse. I also talked to human resources and the engineer was able to assist me in setting up my desk to accommodate my leg being elevated. My coworkers were fabulous. If I needed another chair to elevate my leg, they would grab one to help. They were interested to know how my treatments were going and never made me feel like there was something wrong with me. I also tried not to talk about it too much or draw attention to what I could not do. My goal was to show what I *could* do.

What a Cane Can Do

When patients would see my cane, they were interested to know what had happened. I think it made them feel more connected to me as they knew I was a patient as well as a nurse. By hiring a nurse with a disability, employers are hiring an individual who has experience firsthand in dealing with a disability. This person is an asset to a medical facility, patients, and staff.

My goal was to not have a cane by Christmas 2005. Although I told myself if I was destined to still have it, I decided to make it fun and decorate it with red and white ribbon making it look like I was walking around with a candy cane.

I was very lucky. I found that kind people came out of the woodwork. Many of them had a story to tell or advice to give. When I took the bus, I was welcomed with open arms in the front section of the bus for people with disabilities.

I joined a gym to swim and to do my physical therapy. At the gym, I found a group of people who became my cheerleaders. One woman was a yoga instructor. She volunteered to give me private lessons at no charge. Another friend held my bands every morning and made stretching one of the best times of the day. I took classes in pranic healing. In the class, I met people who provided me a friendship and healing that I will always treasure deeply, and be forever grateful.

I began to find activities that suited my disability. Guitar was one of the new hobbies I acquired. I nurtured my mental health and it led to an inner peace that helped to decrease stress and pain and bring out a creative side I never knew I had.

A Positive, Proactive Approach

I found that you can talk yourself into being sicker than you really are. So I got out of my pajamas and got dressed. I tried to look my best. It made me feel better. It also kept my weight in check (pajamas tend to stretch). I learned to ask for help, too. The doctors were all unable to tell me when and if this would end. I did not want people to get sick of me asking for help or use up all of my favors early on. People generally want to help. But you need to let them know what your needs are (people are not mind readers).

Nurses are natural caretakers, nurturers, and often the caregivers for loved ones. I have never liked feeling vulnerable and dependent on others. I wanted to be the nurse, not the patient. This was a huge life lesson. My friends and family were my support. I will NEVER forget.

For me, it was a time to find out who I really was. I was the traveler, the adventurer. Who was I now? It was a time of introspection and self-exploration. I learned to care for myself and control what I could. I learned not to use my disability as an excuse.

I didn't automatically say "no" to an invitation, and did what I could. Most people do not understand chronic illness, and may stop inviting you if you continue to refuse invitations.

The decision to stay in California and not to return to Australia was one of the hardest I have ever made. But a friend told me about a website called www.Meetup.com. You can search the site for your interest area, and many times you'll find people who share your interest. There happens to be a group of Australians that "meetup" in Los Angeles. I figure if I can't be in Australia, I can join a group full of them.

Also in Los Angeles, a pain management doctor found a recipe that is relieving much of my intense burning pain. I still have pain but I do have relief and my quality of life is greatly improved. I decided to apply at the veterans' hospital. I felt comfortable disclosing my disability and its strengths and limitations. I did not go into great detail. I focused on my abilities as a case manager.

The veterans' hospital hires many people with disabilities and— in my opinion— is the best place I could work. I was hired, and I love my job and the people I work with. After the care the veterans' hospital provided me, I felt the calling to work with other veterans. I have been lucky to care for veterans who served during World War II, the Korean War, Vietnam and the conflicts in Afghanistan and Iraq. Their stories of sacrifice and enthusiasm for life regardless of their losses inspire me on a daily basis. By listening to their stories, it helps me set aside my own problems and focus on what others are going through.

Building Resilience

Find a good doctor

Educate yourself and others

Get out of your pajamas

Ask for help

Keep an open mind

Become your own case manager

Find a support group

Need a cane? Decorate it!

Take care of your mental health

Re-invent yourself

Hold on to your faith

Practice yoga

Play the guitar

Lisa Lobdell, RN, BSN, MSN is a case manager for the veterans' hospital in California. She received her BSN from the California State University Long Beach and her MSN from the University of Phoenix. She can be reached at lisainhawaii@hotmail.com.

Reference

Cluett, J. (2013). *Lisfranc Injury: Fracture-Dislocation of the Midfoot. Retrieved on February 13, 2014 at http://orthopedics.about.com/cs/footproblems/a/lisfranc.htm*

COMMENTARY

By Linda Lang, BA

While some are lucky and find a physician who detects Reflex Sympathetic Dystrophy (RSD) close to its onset, many wait years for a diagnosis. Once entrenched, the disease becomes more complicated and more difficult to deal with. Limbs become more difficult to move, blood flow becomes more restricted, the patient can become more isolated. While this does not mean that remission cannot be achieved, there seems to be a correlation between onset and length of time that treatment begins to how much improvement is achieved.

Over time, the symptoms change. The initial burning pain may calm down while disability may increase. Additionally, a new injury can result in a new site for RSD, which is also called complex regional pain syndrome (CRPS). In these cases, treatment can usually begin quickly enough to be successfully treated.

A (Seemingly) Healthy Exterior

The problem of friends and family not understanding the suffering of the patient or entirely not believing them is very common. We believe in illnesses that can be cured, not in chronic pain that just keeps going. We are also used to seeing someone who is ill and in a great deal of pain manifest the symptoms in their physical appearance: many of those with CRPS look quite healthy.

Some nurses have continued to work after they are diagnosed. Experiences vary from one nurse to the next. I know of one nurse who worked in the NICU. As the pain grew worse, the emotional and physical stress became more than she could handle. A sympathetic supervisor allowed her to cut back on her hours, so she could change her career path. She later went back to school to become a physician's assistant. She got a job in a private doctor's office with reduced stress, shorter hours, and the ability to sit. This worked out quite well for her.

Other nurses, I know, have found switching from a hospital setting to a private physician setting worked better for them. However, several reported their job satisfaction was not as great. Others whose CRPS impacted the upper body were unable to continue to work.

Be honest and ask yourself if you can still perform the duties of a nurse. You then need to ask yourself if anything about your duties or hours can be changed so that you can work more comfortably. Often this may be as easy as cutting back on shifts or the number of hours to your shift. It would also make sense to cut back on your responsibilities at home as the more rest you can get, the better.

Not all jobs come with the ability to adapt to the needs of the employer. Working in a hospital setting probably will not allow the same kind of flexibility as would working for a private physician. Remember, you must be able to perform the duties that fit your job description. While a nurse's job is to treat patients, it is not the employer's job to treat the nurse. So much of workplace success will depend on how severe your CRPS is and how willing you are to push through pain.

Someone with a chronic illness can bring a new understanding to patients in pain and to those patients whose lives will be changed either permanently or temporarily. This is a wonderful asset. Sometimes it may mean changing career paths so that you can concentrate on dealing with the psycho-social rather than the physical side of nursing. Any of these decisions and changes will require a great deal of emotional strength and honesty on your part. It is up to you what you can bring to the table for an employer, not the other way around.

If there is any way you can continue working, you should do it. Feeling useful and fulfilled prevents feelings of hopelessness. It can help take our mind off our own pain, greatly improving both your life and the lives of others.

Choosing whom to tell about your CRPS is tricky, however. If you decide to share the information, it could look like you are asking for special help. It may also make you feel self-conscious—thinking others are looking over your shoulder to make sure you are not "slacking off." Share as little information as possible if you want to be treated the same as anyone else. While you may feel especially close to one colleague and may want to share what you are going through, telling one is often the same as telling all. Save your sharing for your friends at home.

Once you have had time to adapt emotionally to your diagnosis and find that treatment is helping you overcome many physical problems, you may want to proudly tell your colleagues what you have been able to overcome and educate them about CRPS. Who knows when one of their patients will have the disease?

Search for Information

Find out what other nurses have written about the problem. Search the nursing literature for information. Consider writing about your experiences as a nurse who happens to have CRPS. Set up a private Facebook page and invite others like yourself to share their experiences. Establish relationships with groups like www.ExceptionalNurse.com and start a conversation with other nurses.

Also, consider starting a support group. The Reflex Sympathetic Dystrophy Association can help you with that by giving you a forum. Through a support group, you can get help from others thinking about employment settings and practice roles that facilitate continued employment. You can also discuss accommodations that employers make for nurses, and include the emotional benefits to nurses as well as the hidden pitfalls.

Once you have identified enough nurses, consider fundraising events both to educate the public and finance some of the things you want to accomplish. Remember no matter what you decide, you must first take care of yourself and conserve your strength for what matters most. Pick and choose your battles. The Reflex Sympathetic Dystrophy Association (www.rsds.org) will support you in any way it can.

Linda Lang, B.A. is author of Living with RSDS: Your Guide to Coping with Reflex Sympathetic Dystrophy Syndrome. *She is a board member of the Reflex Sympathetic Dystrophy Association* / index2.html

Suggested Reading

Lang, L. & Moskowitz, P. (2003). *Living with RSDS: Your Guide to Coping with Reflex Sympathetic Dystrophy Syndrome*, CA: New Harbinger Publications.

11 PROVING MYSELF OVER AND OVER: NURSING WITH HEARING LOSS AND A COCHLEAR IMPLANT

By Linda J. Keyes, RN, BS

Ever since I was a child, I knew I wanted to be a nurse or work in a profession that involved interaction with people. As a young child, I spent several months in a hospital due to illness. I interacted with doctors, nurses, audiologists, hearing aid specialists, and so forth. I was destined to work with people and "give back" what was given to me. I remember being inquisitive and asking lots of questions about "how" and "why" things worked within the body.

At four years of age, I was diagnosed with a profound, moderate hearing loss. My mother contracted rubella while carrying me in utero. Because I read lips so well, I fooled others for a long period of time. It was discovered in preschool when I did not turn to answer a teacher who called my name. My parents purchased a set of bi-cross hearing aids and I began my journey.

Daring Me to Succeed

In high school, a teacher said, "You will never make it as a registered nurse." That was just the *drive* I needed to do it! In junior high school, I was told I could not take a language because of my hearing loss. I was deeply disappointed and *vowed* that I would never be told "no" ever again. The first class I took in college was Spanish and I received an "A." It gave me even stronger wings. Little did I know that I was going to have to "prove" myself over and over again— it would not be a "one-time deal."

I attended the BSN program at the University of Connecticut from 1983 until 1985. I completed some of my prerequisite courses for nursing but decided a smaller school would be a better fit for someone with hearing loss, so I transferred to Baystate Medical Center School of Nursing in Springfield, MA. How excited I was at this point in my life!

Accommodations in nursing school included an amplified

128

stethoscope (a big clunky thing that looked more like a stethoscope from barbaric times!), sitting up front in class, and comparing notes with other students or even photocopying the notes to ensure that I had all the correct information. I had meetings with faculty to make sure my accommodations were appropriate and if I had any questions that needed clarification. The faculty was fantastic in terms of support. I could not have asked for more.

However, in March of 1986, I found my confidence wavering in clinical when a surgeon was upset because a staple remover was not at the patient's bedside. The nurses on the floor said they had run out of them and they would try to get one right away. The surgeon was disgruntled and verbally abusive. I passed out at the bedside due to the stress of the situation. I began to think the hearing loss was the reason for my confidence wavering and considered leaving nursing school. I remembered I *was* told once I would not be able to be a nurse.

Having to Leave

After deep thought, I decided I was not ready to face the doctors who were demeaning to others and needed to leave nursing school. I gave my resignation despite the dean encouraging me to stay. I was simply not willing to be treated this way and saddened by this discovery. Thinking of what others were thinking of me with my bulky stethoscope and my confidence wavering, I felt it was time to try another avenue. I did promise myself that one day, I would return to nursing school when I regained my confidence.

I returned to the University of Connecticut majoring in family studies, and decided I would become a therapist. However, I was still torn between nursing and therapy, so I combined my internships doing work that included therapy and nursing. I lived on campus, adjusted to college life and graduated in December of 1988 with a degree in human development and family relations. It was not long after this, I decided I wanted to return to nursing school to prove to myself I could, indeed become a nurse.

Back to Nursing

In 1990, I re-entered Baystate Medical Center School of Nursing. The faculty that remained from my first enrollment were thrilled to witness my return! The greetings were warm and welcoming. Returning to nursing school felt like a breeze this time. I had simply matured and it no longer mattered what people thought about my disability. I worked as an aide in labor and delivery in the evenings and attended school during the day. I sailed through until my medical-surgical rotation, where I encountered a very difficult nursing professor whom I felt simply did not want me to become an RN. She tried numerous times to fail me. Needless to say, I prevailed.

Then I came down with the chicken pox. When I returned to school, I had to complete two med-surg exams on Monday, two on Tuesday, an oral presentation on Thursday, and a term paper was due on Friday. I have no idea how I managed but through the grace of God, I did.

On graduation in June 1993, I was one of the first two people to get hired as a new graduate nurse. At that time, jobs were scarce. I began my nursing career as a new graduate on a medical-surgical unit in a small community hospital in Connecticut. I took my nursing boards later that summer and passed. I made my own accommodations at this point. A state vocational rehabilitation counselor assisted me in purchasing an amplified stethoscope— one that required taking my hearing aids out to use it.

A Supportive Team

The supervisors knew I had a hearing loss, but it was never an issue. I was a visual learner and my co-workers were fantastic to work with. I had a charge nurse whom I will always be grateful to for serving as my mentor. An excellent nurse herself, she taught the new graduates well. She was strict and stern but the patient's safety and best interest was always paramount. Years later, she shared with me that I was a very intuitive nurse and could pick up on things that were taking place with the patients. Sometimes, it was just simply gut intuition. I have had this gift most of my life. I continued in medical-surgical nursing for five years. Then, my colleagues suggested that I consider ICU nursing. They felt that I would do very well there.

So soon I found myself working in ICU. It was a wonderful

experience—scary but a new learning environment. I found it easier to work in ICU due to the smaller size and circular shape of the unit. You could see every room from any point from the nursing station. There were alarms I had to learn to recognize, ventilators, call bells, IV pumps, and cardiac monitors. I continued to work with few accommodations.

But I had to work with many physicians who were Indian and they had heavy accents. That was my biggest challenge. I clearly remember apologizing to a cardiologist, "I am sorry. It is very hard for me to understand you. I have a hearing loss and sometimes it is difficult for me to understand."

I'll never forget his kind words, "Linda, please don't be sorry. I have a very heavy accent. It takes two of us to work together to make it work." It was the most positive feedback I'd heard from a physician. From that day on, we did work together.

My colleagues would assist if a procedure was done with masks that would prevent me from reading lips. They would step in when needed and assist me or we would trade. Another nurse might have needed to do a dressing change and I would do the dressing change and he or she would assist with a procedure that required wearing masks—central line placements— were a particular challenge. Once I learned the steps of the line placements and the personalities of the doctors, I adapted very well.

During this time, there were no issues with colleagues or administration, and I received excellent evaluations. I continued in ICU for approximately four more years; and then in a medical-surgical unit for a year. I loved the hospice on that unit. Eventually, I returned to ICU and remained torn between the two places I loved to be.

A Sudden Change

In January of 2003, a turn of events completely changed my life. While at work one morning just before shift change, suddenly everyone sounded to me as if they had a stroke— their speech was garbled and I could not understand the staff. My gut told me "this is not a wax in my ears problem"…sounds funny today but it was not so funny at the time.

I ended up going to see eight doctors, and in a matter of two days, my hearing was gone. Seven of the doctors told me, "Your hearing is gone, you need to go sign up with the receptionist for an appointment to be evaluated for a cochlear implant." They also added, "You will no longer be able to practice nursing."

I thought to myself, "My life is over."

There were many, many days of tears. Finally, I met a surgeon in Boston who *really* listened and saw my grief. He said, "I am not going to tell you to get a cochlear implant but I will recommend that you consider it." He also shared, "You will NOT have to give up nursing. I have implanted two nurses and a physician and they are doing very well."

In the meantime, while waiting in the waiting room, I met another nurse who lost her hearing overnight. Both of us were so grief stricken with our losses. She had lost her job, too.

In the meantime, I was placed on short- then long-term disability. My implant surgery was scheduled in June. I remember begging to work at the hospital. I asked if I could even work as an aide. The response was, "But aides need their hearing."

Also, I was told my insurance benefits were going to cease. I informed them of federal laws regarding COBRA. I even asked about other jobs in social services but a representative in human resources admitted to forgetting to check into them.

I lost my job and was unemployed for two years. I went everywhere and any place I could think of— refusing to give up as a nurse. Finally, I ended up volunteering at a local community college nursing program helping in a simulation lab with their nursing students. It was a new beginning for me.

The dean of the school suggested, "I think you should apply to this nursing home for a job." It was very disheartening—a former ICU nurse working in a nursing home? But, I followed her advice and went to work at the nursing home. I did paperwork for Medicare reimbursement. While I was grateful for a job, I can tell you that I cried every single day to and from work. In addition, my significant other left after three-and-a-half years together. I remember asking God, "Ok, here's the deal: I will do whatever you want me to do but you have to promise me that things will get better."

A few months later, I started floor nursing at the nursing home in acute rehab. I was faced with working with some very demeaning licensed practical nurses. It was grueling work, but I made a promise to God to keep my end of the bargain. The nurses were not accommodating in assisting me to use the telephone for orders. I asked a charge nurse if she could please place a call to the doctor for me and I was asked why, and I informed her that my patient's blood pressure was in the 70's/40's and he was a full code. She said, "Oh, that's ok, you can leave a note on the desk for the doctor when he comes in on Monday."

This is the treatment I endured. I learned not to listen to others and to stay with my gut instincts, and keep my promise to God.

A Rocky But Manageable Road

At this point, I had to have three cochlear implant surgeries due to complications. I spent two years rehabilitating my hearing, trying to re-establish a career and restoring my soul. It was challenging to say the least. I had been hired by a hospital and the start date was delayed for 15 months due to an employee health nurse who would not release me to work.

Despite providing education, documentation, references from the literature and contacts, it was futile. Everyone else was agreeable and looking forward to having me work with them, including the director of nursing in cardiology and the medical director. Ironically, this very hospital did one of my cochlear implant surgeries.

The employee health nurse wanted my accommodations in writing and signed before I started. The problem was, not knowing all of the accommodations that I would need prior to starting the position. It was a difficult battle and mainly due to one nurse.

In the meantime, I heard from a small community hospital in

Massachusetts. I was interviewed by two RN's. I made it very clear to them that if having cochlear implants was an issue for them, to please let me know NOW because I did not want to waste their time or mine. My tolerance had grown to almost zero at this point. The supervisor smiled and said, "It is not a problem for us. We would love to have you work with us."

So, from that point on, I was back in the hospital. I worked on a medical-surgical unit for about a year and then transferred to ICU. I floated there one day and was noticed by the director for my patient care. On the medical surgical unit, I was fairly well-received although there were the occasional looks I got at times when I asked someone to repeat what they said.

My boss was absolutely one of the best directors I ever worked for. She had no tolerance for discrimination. I did feel it from some co-workers but I let it go. It was too much of a risk to make an issue of it. I was back in the saddle and that is where I wanted to stay!

After transferring to ICU, I worked there for about nine months and had a calling to move to Colorado. I decided it was time to spread my wings. I left New England and began my journey in Colorado. I worked in ICU for two-and-a-half years and have recently started working in an inpatient hospice. I really liked what I was doing in ICU but the passion was waning. So, I needed to follow my heart.

Ironically, my life came full circle. I was able to return to my nursing career despite all of the odds. It saddened me deeply and profoundly when I lost my original job. But now when I look back on it, my life would not be where it is today. Keeping up my credentials and volunteering were important parts of my success. And there are a few people that I owe much, much gratitude for their role in my journey. If it wasn't for the support of my family, my dog, Sadie, and my friends, I would never have made it. Life is good!

Special thanks to my vocational rehabilitation counselors and organizations like www.ExceptionalNurse.com, and www.Amphl. If it were not for these people, and organizations, the road would have been so much more difficult!

Building Resilience

Step out of nursing school or nursing practice, if needed

Take time to heal or regain confidence

Get back on the horse as soon as possible

Volunteer

Keep up your credentials

Find the right lane to swim in

Give thanks to all who helped along the way

Linda Keyes, RN, works for Exempla Lutheran Medical Center in Wheatridge, CO. She lives in Castle Rock, CO, and can be reached at ljkeyes93@yahoo.com

COMMENTARY

By Marcia Kolvitz, PhD

"What will you be when you grow up?" is a common question that young children are asked. The answers are often accompanied by advice for the student about the best course of action to meet that goal, opinions about job opportunities in that field, or even comments about how good of a "match" that student might (or might not) be for that profession. Many young people, however, have limited exposure to the vast array of career opportunities available to them and even less information about what it might take to be successful in a particular field.

Role models can be extremely helpful in helping the student create a vision for his or her future. Since hearing loss is often described as an "invisible disability," students who are deaf or hard of hearing may not have had the opportunity to observe or interact with professionals with hearing loss during the career exploration process. Although there are nurses who are deaf or hard of hearing currently working in various settings, they represent only a small portion of the entire population of nurses. Despite the dearth of role models, there's a growing group of young adults who are exploring the possibility of careers in healthcare and asking, "Why not?"

Reports continue to circulate regarding the current nursing shortage and the anticipated increased need for nurses in the future (American Association of Colleges of Nursing, 2014). Organizations, including the Association of Medical Professionals with Hearing Losses (AMPHL), support tapping into the available pool of qualified and motivated individuals to increase the number and diversity of nurses entering and remaining in the field.

Although some people may ask, "How can someone with a hearing loss become a nurse?" the experiences of students with hearing loss can vary significantly among individuals. A number of personal and environmental factors will have an impact on how the student learns and how he or she interacts with instructors, peers, and patients. Other factors include degree of hearing loss, age of onset of hearing loss, and educational background. Ambient noise levels, room acoustics, and lighting also can have a significant impact on how well communication might flow between a health care provider and a patient.

Instead of focusing on what someone with a hearing loss cannot do, why not consider strategies to create a more welcoming environment? In many settings, simple changes can be made that may benefit more than just one person. Using the principles of universal design, adding visual signals such as flashing lights in addition to auditory signals can alert any member of the staff. Using pagers is a common way of communicating, and it creates a more accessible work environment for everyone.

Planning for the Future

Before committing to any program or major area of study, students should understand as much about themselves as possible. Do you like to work with people or do you prefer to work alone? Are you interested in science and not squeamish in hospital settings or when around blood or other body fluids? Can you remain calm and organized when handling emergency situations? Career interest inventories can assist students in discovering what jobs they would find most interesting. Career aptitude tests can help students better understand their aptitudes or talents.

The Postsecondary Education Programs Network (PEPNet) offers a variety of online resources to assist students in preparing for postsecondary education and training. PEPNet is funded through a cooperative agreement with the U.S. Department of Education, Office of Special Education Programs; its mission is to improve transition services and educational access for students who are deaf or hard of hearing.

Many young adults can benefit from knowing that peers have had similar experiences and created successful lives. Having role models and mentors can be a valuable experience when considering options for the future. To address this, PEPNet developed a series of publications and videos that might be of interest to teenagers and young adults.

Communication Access

Many students enroll in college and utilize the same types of services that they used throughout their education: sign language interpreters, assistive listening devices, oral interpreters, note takers, or captioning services. Others find that what worked in high school might not be as effective for them in college. Students considering careers in nursing will also need to consider how effective communication access can be provided in clinical settings.

Students who need additional visual cues for classroom access may request speech-to-text services, sign language interpreters, or oral interpreters. Speech-to-text service providers (often referred to as a captioner or transcriber) use specialized software and a display device to provide a text format of the lecture and discussion. Students who use sign language interpreters should discuss the preferred mode of communication (e.g., use of American Sign Language or use of Contact Sign), review terminology, and establish what signs could be used to express specific concepts for each class. Students with strong speech reading skills may request an oral interpreter. An oral interpreter will present on the lips and face what is being said during the conversation or presentation.

Many students use personal hearing aids to understand speech and detect environmental cues. Although hearing aid technology has improved tremendously over the past few decades, there are limitations to how strong the signal might be. Older analog hearing aids tend to amplify all sounds, making it difficult to separate background noise from speech; the sound produced by newer digital hearing aids is clearer and has reduced distortion and internal noise. High-end digital hearing aids may also be programmed for different listening situations. Purchasing and maintaining a personal hearing aid is the student's responsibility. Assistive listening devices (ALD) amplify the speaker's voice and reduce the influence of background noise. Commonly used ALDs include FM systems, infrared systems, and electromagnetic induction loop systems. Because an ALD might be used by several different students, this equipment is generally purchased and maintained by the institution.

In the college environment, students who are deaf or hard of hearing are strongly encouraged to take an active role in planning their communication access services. Discussions with the staff in the disability services office can be helpful prior to the start of a new term, especially when the student's course load includes laboratory work or clinical assignments. Service providers, such as interpreters or speech-to-text providers, may need to prepare for the terminology used in the classes or work with the student to determine the best sight lines to see the access service, the instructor, and any visual course materials used.

In clinical settings, students will be expected to identify heart, lung, and bowel sounds; communicate in settings in which surgical masks are used; and communicate with patients in a clinical setting or on the telephone. Students with hearing loss may not be able to utilize a traditional acoustic stethoscope. Several amplified stethoscope models are available, and students who benefit from hearing aids are encouraged to work with faculty and their audiologist to determine a good match. Technology such as text pagers and smartphones can be an effective strategy for handling alerts and telephone messages. There are numerous materials available on the PEPNet website that may provide a student with additional information: www.pepnet.org.

Marcia Kolvitz, PhD, is the Director, PEPNet-South at The University of Tennessee, Knoxville.

References

American Association of Colleges of Nursing (2014). Nursing shortage (fact sheet).
http://www.aacn.nche.edu/Media/FactSheets/NursingShortage.htm

Postsecondary Education Programs Network (PEPNet). www.pepnet.org

Suggested Reading

Association of Medical Professionals with Hearing Losses
www.amphl.org

UK Health Professionals with Hearing Loss

http://hphl.org.uk/links/health-professionals-with-hearing-loss

Understanding stethoscopes

http://pepnet.org/sites/default/files/129understanding%20stethosco
pe%20FAQ.pdf

12 ONE STRAW TOO MANY: NURSING THROUGH BLOOD CLOTS, DEPRESSION, AND HURRICANE HUGO

By Margot Withrow, RN, BSN, CCRN as told to John Owen, MA

At about the age of four, I knew I wanted to become a nurse. In high school, I excelled in science, math, and biology, and graduated with vocational honors. Through a weekend program at the local technical college, I became a certified nursing assistant and learned CPR through the local fire department. All the while, I worked at a "Stop and Shop" store.

Placement tests for the nursing program at the nearby community college revealed that my reading scores weren't high enough. So, during my first year, I took remedial reading and most of my electives. I graduated in three years with my associate's degree in nursing.

I was assigned to take my boards in Raleigh, NC. It was my first time in a big city and I was filled with fear of failure— I even broke out in hives—but I passed! It was 1984, a time without a nursing shortage. Still working flexible hours at the store, I got the opportunity to fill in nights and weekends working intermediate care at a nursing home. Later, I moved to full time on the skilled floor.

I moved on to gain hospital experience, working on telemetry and medical-surgical floors at a local hospital while still working shifts at the nursing home. Then I got sick with blood clots: a pulmonary embolus and left leg deep vein thrombophlebitis. I had an occluded vein and risked throwing a clot, so I was put on 14 days strict bed rest. I turned 22 years old in the hospital. I missed six weeks of work. The doctor released me for "light duty"— but there was no such thing at my job.

In 1988, I moved to Chapel Hill to pursue my BSN at the University of North Carolina. Along with school, I was working 20-hour days—I lasted just three months due to the stress. Only when I went in to resign was I offered help and counseling, but it was too late. I had to borrow money to cover my broken lease and my moving expenses. I was filled with depression and a deep sense of failure. Within two weeks, I was back to work PRN at my old hospital.

Hurricane Hugo Arrives

At a friend's suggestion, I became a travel nurse and moved to South Carolina. I was recruited to a hospital in Charleston. I started on Monday with an eight-hour orientation and Hurricane Hugo hit that Thursday. When the storm started to make the news the day before, my dad called and urged me to come back home, but I felt I couldn't "desert the ship." The travel company said they couldn't ask us to stay and risk our lives, but made a verbal promise of a $1,000 bonus if we stayed and worked. I stocked up on Sternos and Vienna sausages.

When I went to work Thursday morning, it was raining "cats and dogs." I worked 12 hours, then took a cold shower in an operating room and went to catch some sleep in a converted room on a hospital ward. The windows were taped to prevent shattering. Transformers popped like fireworks and cars were floating in the water.

In the moment before the power went out, the TV announced that Hugo was here. The windows blew out, and I moved to the hallway fighting back panic. The backup generators took over. While sitting in a wheelchair in the hall with my head against the wall, I could feel the steel beams moving. I felt I was going to die—oddly peaceful.

An elderly woman coded. The elevators were out and she had to be carried up four flights of steps as emergency response continued. The unit was crazy. Ventilators cut on and off. The patients had to be manually bagged by lay staff and therapists.

In 40 hours, I had maybe 20 minutes sleep and had to face another 12-hour shift. The lab had flooded and the ICU had no windows. The head nurse hadn't made it in due to the weather, so as the RN, I was in charge of the ICU with six patients, all on ventilators. Of the other two licensed practical nurses, one had no ICU experience and the other had forgotten her blood pressure medicine.

The septic system had backed up and the smell was awful. I wondered constantly what I had forgotten to do... And then a freshly showered resident turned up asking for labs. I wondered where he had been.

By Friday, the hospital had run low on food but the roads were said to be passable. Trees were down and the National Guard was out. It was like a warzone. I felt addled and disoriented. I was off for the weekend.

While the hospital had generators, my apartment was without power for three weeks. Some weeks later the travel company sent a letter of commendation thanking all who had stayed and risked their lives. The bonus was only $100.

After the Storm

In April, I began seeing a therapist weekly, at first for weight issues but later with a diagnosis of depression and PTSD. I did this on my own dime, picking up extra shifts to cover. I had survivor's guilt and often second-guessed myself, not to mention suffering anxiety in thunderstorms. My insurance didn't cover the therapy. Because of the stigma associated with mental health issues, I feared losing my job if I were to tell anyone.

An opportunity for a promotion and chance to go back to school fell through, so I jumped to yet another hospital. I worked there for the next nine years, obtained critical care registered nurse certification (CCRN), and finally got the chance to finish my BSN. I got up at 5:00 a.m., commuted 50 miles to work, took classes from 8:00 a.m. to 4:00 p.m., and then worked a 12-hour shift before driving home the next morning. By May of 1994, I had my BSN degree.

Then I began to work a modified Baylor: six shifts in 14 days with some overtime. I worked the ICU and floated to telemetry when the census dropped. During this time, I suffered clots twice and was out for six weeks; three times with superficial phlebitis. Again, my doctor ordered "light duty," but there was no such thing. I felt helpless and afraid of losing my job. Since my twenties, I realized I had a pre-existing condition with the clots and was fearful of jumping jobs, plus I was vested in the retirement plan, so I felt like I couldn't move on.

I was only scheduled as a charge nurse with the most inexperienced teams, perhaps in an effort to force me out. I often asked to be taken off that duty. My requests were denied so I transferred to the psychiatric unit.

After an orientation to the psychiatric unit, I became increasingly concerned with my weight gain, always having leaned towards the heavy side. I quit my Prozac and ordered some Meridia online, and tried some hypnosis tapes for weight loss. Rather than lose, I showed rapid weight gain. I consulted a psychiatrist I worked with and began another antidepressant. I became paranoid and increasingly labile.

Spiraling Out of Control

My parents came to take me home. Later, I got into a fight with my mother and trashed the house. I was taken by ambulance in face-down restraints to the local ER, and then transferred involuntarily to the state mental hospital I had worked at years before. I was held in seclusion, had restraints and was heavily sedated. By the time I was released, I had gained even more weight and also had lymphedema. I suspect I may have had signs of neuroleptic malignant syndrome.

I fell on to the disability rolls; doubly depressed at the loss of my career, which had been the center of my life. By 2006, I was in a suicidal depression. I was diabetic and in and out of the state and local mental hospitals. I developed problems with lithium toxicity and became insulin dependent. My health situation just became more and more complicated.

One sustaining factor during these difficult times was becoming aware of the mental health advocacy movement within the state. I began to accept my life and try to live by the three Cs: I did not *cause* the situation, I cannot

change the situation, and I cannot *cure* the situation.
Rather than dwell on my failures, I'm trying to embrace positive aspects of myself.

Only in the last year, have I begun to realize that while my working career as a nurse came to an end in 2001, I am and always will be a nurse with or without my license, employed or not. Only recently, have I realized that I worked as a nurse with a disability all along. Because of blood clots, I had been on blood thinners all that time. And I suffered through depression and post-traumatic stress.

A nurse works a lot of hours, puts off the need to void, misses meals in favor of crackers and a gulp of soda to push through those 12-hour shifts, knowing the next one is not going to be any easier. I had planned to work until age 70, but went out at age 37. I am living proof you can nurse yourself almost to death.

After admission to the state mental hospital, I was given no hope of ever recovering or in any way getting back on my feet. For years, I was kept overmedicated. Through it all, I kept up my continuing education and my license; but am dependent now on disability for my health coverage and medications.

Find Your Worth Outside of Career

Having built my self-esteem on my profession, it has been a struggle to recover it. One lesson here is not to make your job your life, because in the normal course of events you can lose the one before the other. Hindsight reminds me that outside activities and a life outside the constraints of the profession are important to achieving balance in life.

Looking back, I may have worked too hard and said "no" all too rarely. I didn't stop to take care of myself, even as I put all my energy into caring for my patients. And the system did nothing to support or stop me. After a major hurricane, there was no crisis intervention and debriefing. There was virtually no allowance for human frailty.

Nursing, especially hospital nursing, may be a unique profession in that shifts must be staffed 24/7, 365 days a year. Lengthy shifts and hours that would be decried as sweatshop labor in other professions are a norm. On one hand, long-term policy change might call for shift reform to regulate the unreasonable demands on nursing staff, but until that day comes, nurses should confront the realities in orientation to nursing school and be taught the importance of looking after themselves.

It is impossible to care for others if you fail to care for yourself. A nurse must learn to say no. Even the airlines say put on your own oxygen mask before putting one on someone else. The importance of self-care and self-assessment need to be stressed right from the start.

Nursing can physically or mentally break the worker. As nurses fall out of the profession, a new class graduates and is ready to take their place. Realistic career planning that encompasses a range of possibilities should start in nursing school.

Employee assistance programs (EAPs) might be a valuable resource to some people, but in my experience, they have trouble living up to their promise. For one thing, although they are supposed to be confidential, word would often get out that an employee was going there. And all too often, the counseling would reportedly not live up to the demands. Still the EAP might be a base to build on for counseling nurses who show signs of stress illnesses, mental health problems, or on-the-job conflict.

Mandatory debriefing should be required after especially stressful situations. Given the realities of double shifting and extra hours, team debriefings may seem like a luxury, but should become part of the routine. Nurses confront death, illness, injury and disfigurement face to face on a daily basis, and nothing is gained by turning the blind eye of denial to such harsh, cold facts of the stress of being a nurse. Caregivers also need care. And after a disaster, such as a major hurricane, crisis intervention teams should not overlook the caregiving professions.

Remove the Stigma of Mental Illness

Finally, a word must be said about the stigma attached to disability in the nursing profession and to mental illness in society as a whole. It is only in retrospect that I realized I had worked with a disability most of my career. In many ways, dealing with blood clots brought out my stubborn can-do side. I may have been overcompensating in a drive to prove I was as well as the next person and as capable of doing my job.

Because depression never made me miss a day's work or fail to get out of bed at whatever hour was necessary, I may have denied its power over me. And without my job, I feel my depression would have possibly been worse: Everyone needs a meaningful day.

Given social attitudes, I may well have failed to admit to myself that in addition to the obvious blood clots, I had a mental illness. And beyond seeing a therapist, I knew nothing of the possible supports out in the world for such problems.

Mental illness needs to be brought out from the cloud of shame and denial in order for it to be addressed as an issue. An invisible disability may well be one of the trickiest issues under the Americans with Disabilities Act. Disclosure could easily trigger covert discrimination.

Nurses need accurate mental health self-assessments and a willingness to seek help preventively. By the time a nurse gets written up for a workplace situation, it may already be both too late to obtain an accommodation and to get needed help. Don't wait until it is too late. Some nurses I worked with lost their licenses to drugs or their lives to suicide. And sometimes I'm left feeling like the walking wounded myself.

With support though, I'm beginning to see I've achieved much in the face of adversity and should hold my head up. Once a nurse, always a nurse.

Building Resilience

Take care of yourself

Include a wide range of options in career planning

Consider EAP programs and disclosure cautiously

Seek help when needed

Hold your head high

Margot Withrow, R.N., B.S.N., CCRN enjoys knitting, handcrafts, and the company of her cat, Midnite. She is currently being medically re-evaluated. She still maintains her nursing license and CEUs. She can be reached at margot_withrow@yahoo.com

John Owen, M.A., has two longstanding incompletes on his Yale J.D. and past experience in the Yale Disability Law Clinic. He does volunteer work as a mental health consumer advocate on the state and local levels, currently serving on the North Carolina Commission on Mental Health, Developmental Disabilities, and Substance Abuse. He can be reached at jolesowen@gmail.com.

COMMENTARY

By John S. Murray, PhD, RN, CPNP, CS, FAAN

Recent natural and man-made disasters such as the catastrophic F5 tornado in Moore, Oklahoma, and the Colorado wildfires to the Boston marathon bombings, remind us how disasters can strike without notice and with little time for preparation. Nurses have been long recognized for their significant contributions to disaster response, frequently placing their own health and safety secondary to relief efforts. Often there is no time to contemplate what challenges might be faced as a result of being an essential responder. In fact, little attention is given to the physical and mental health demands as well as potential legal and ethical challenges nurses may face during and after catastrophic events.

As articulately described by the authors, nurses responding to disasters face a number of demanding challenges. Often health care institutions are overwhelmed by the rapid escalation in demand for resources to the point of services being brought to a standstill. Frequently, only minimal staff is available to work and do so under austere conditions and extraordinary stress. Equipment is often inoperable as power supplies are nonexistent. Simple amenities such as working toilets, running water, air conditioning, and operating elevators are commonly unavailable during disasters.

From a psychological perspective, there is a collective sense of fear and panic among healthcare staff, patients, families, and visitors. When lines of communication outside the healthcare organization are cut off, mass confusion ensues, which has the potential to erode the psyche of staff. These emotions are intensified by long and unpredictable hours worked, extended periods of moving patients, heavy equipment, and supplies to safer locations within the healthcare institution, and providing manual ventilation to patients as described by the authors.

When working conditions become more extreme as supplies and resources dwindle, it is not uncommon for nurses to struggle with the ethical concern of being unable to provide care to every patient. While disaster responders are trained to provide the greatest good for the greatest number, during extreme conditions this may feel like a daunting task. For example, how are food, water, medications, and supplies rationed? Who gets treated first? These are ethical questions, which received great attention in the aftermath of Hurricane Katrina.

Nurses must recognize that not every need will be met during a disaster. However, it is important for them to remember that despite what level of care they are able to provide, it is possible to treat all patients with respect and dignity especially in situations and decisions regarding life and death.

Another concern that arises for nurses is the potential legal implications of responding during disasters. Hurricane Katrina, more than any other disaster, highlighted legal concerns that may be faced by healthcare professionals. Most nurses questioned if their nursing license was protected and wondered what assurance was in place to prevent malpractice lawsuits when they were required to provide care under severe circumstances. This continues to be an area requiring additional debate by professional organizations and disaster planners.

The aforementioned issues nurses faced in disaster were previously due, in part, to a lack of guidelines for healthcare professionals during catastrophes. Disaster experts have long recognized that a framework is needed to provide guidance to healthcare professionals regarding expectations and legal protections during disasters where altered standards of care occur. Over the past couple of years, the American Nurses Association and other professional organizations have worked collaboratively to address the need for effective policies and plans for disaster preparedness and response so that staff has an awareness of their expected role during disasters.

Disaster Response Guidelines

In 2012, the Institute of Medicine published guidelines (Crisis Standards of Care) offering a rigorous systems framework for providing disaster response. The framework ensures that healthcare professionals responding to disasters do so following consistent protocols which also take into consideration the ethical and legal concerns related to caring for individuals during catastrophic events. Those who have invested time into developing the crisis standards of care for catastrophic events hope that this framework will provide the guidance, confidence in decision making, and responses to the ethical and legal concerns health care personnel have related to disaster response.

Undoubtedly, nurses responding to disasters must be supported in addressing their concerns related to disasters during and following response efforts. Appropriate plans necessary to guide practice under stressful and austere conditions are critically important. Hospital administrators, chief nursing officers, and organization emergency preparedness coordinators have a responsibility to ensure crisis standards of care are available to staff. All nurses should familiarize themselves with these resources to optimize disaster response so everyone is best prepared to meet the needs of those affected by devastating events. (Free online access to Crisis Standards of Care can be found at:

http://www.iom.edu/Reports/2012/Crisis-Standards-of-Care-A-Systems-Framework-for-Catastrophic-Disaster-Response.aspx).

Just as important, the disaster response community needs to acknowledge ongoing mental healthcare may be needed for some responders. Individuals experience a range of emotional responses which can be temporary or long lasting. Disaster response involves exposure to an extreme, traumatic stressor, which should be monitored over an extended period of time with behavioral health support provided as needed for those who courageously respond to disasters. It is vital to use all appropriate endeavors to prevent the development of chronic and disabling problems such as post-traumatic stress disorder, depression, and substance use and misuse.

John S. Murray, PhD, RN, CPNP, CS, FAAN has served in a variety of leadership, clinical, education and research positions in both military and civilian healthcare systems. He has written over 60 peer-reviewed journal articles and five book chapters including articles related to public health emergencies, responding to the psychosocial needs of children and families in disasters, disaster preparedness for children with special health care needs and disabilities and frameworks for responding to catastrophic events. Dr. Murray is the past contributing editor, Disaster Care, American Journal of Nursing. He can be reached at jmurray325@aol.com.

Suggested Reading

Murray, J.S. (2012). Crisis standards of care: A framework for responding to catastrophic disasters. What the new IOM guidelines mean for nurses. *American Journal of Nursing, 112*(10), 65-67.

Murray, J.S. (2012). National Disaster Medical System: Providing disaster care of national significance. What the new IOM guidelines mean for nurses. *American Journal of Nursing, 112*(2), 65-70.

13 TOUGH TIMES DON'T LAST, BUT TOUGH PEOPLE DO: NURSING AFTER A LOWER LIMB AMPUTATION

By Carolyn McKinzie, LPN

It's hard to know how to prepare yourself mentally when faced with amputation. I am a fairly smart person, but I felt dumb. All of my nursing knowledge seemed to have disappeared when I became the patient facing a huge unknown. That day of my amputation, I didn't have the slightest clue about anything. I was full of questions: How could this happen to me? What had I ever done to deserve so much agony and pain? I felt helpless and alone. It had been such a long and difficult struggle since my car accident two-and-a-half years prior. I felt so tired: my body, my mind, and my soul.

My spirit was totally gone. I had nothing left. I didn't want to fight it anymore. I was absolutely exhausted from this journey. I wanted to give up, to throw in the towel, and say the hell with it all. I just didn't care anymore. I felt as though I had lost such a big part of myself, much more than just a leg.

There was a possibility that this day might come, but I had been optimistic after the last surgery. It had been successful and the leg stayed healed for more than a year. It was the longest time following a surgery that the leg had healed and stayed together for more than just a few weeks. But there was always that lingering knowledge in the back of my mind that anything could happen. It would only take a split second to undo any amount of the repair, and if that happened, it would be the end.

I had tried conservation therapy nearly a dozen times after the initial auto accident in October 1998 and a fall in February 2001 and the reality of starting all of that over again was frightening at best. I tried not to dwell on that and I tried to remain positive. I relived all that I had been through over the years and months leading up to this point. Sometimes even *I* marveled at my progress. I was lucky to have my leg for as long as I did. I knew that I had the best surgeons, and everything that could have been done to save the leg had been done. They did all they could and then some; the healing was up to me and me alone.

A Different Outcome

So here I was, again faced with a relapse. It was different this time. The previous surgeries were all done with the intent to heal and solidify the fracture; healing was always the anticipated outcome, but not this time. This time it was more definitive and I knew what the end result would be. I felt like I had lost the final battle. I had fought so hard, and did everything I could to allow my body to heal. I never gave up.

I felt sad this time like I was losing a friend; I was grieving. Sure, it was just a leg, but it had so much history and I had been through so much because of it. It would be hard to let go of it emotionally. I wasn't just losing my leg; I was losing a part of my life. I cried every day for weeks. Some days I cried *all* day, some days, just a few times. The time before my surgery seemed like an eternity.

I wondered what would become of me. How much rehabilitation would it take and to what degree would I recover. What if I didn't have the physical or emotional strength to recover enough to regain my mobility? I pictured myself, bedridden, like an old woman, and I feared that life as I knew it would soon be over. I couldn't imagine ever smiling again, or laughing, or even wanting to for that matter. I knew my career was gone. All that I had put into my life's work over the years was gone and I would never be able to get that back.

Lacking Purpose

I wondered what my purpose in life really was. Before all of this, it had been my nursing, I thought. But now what? That was gone forever, I thought. I felt that my purpose in life was to be doing something beneficial to others and I believed that was the reason I had been spared from death in the accident. I was needed here; I had much more work to do, but now all of that had changed. I felt like I had sunk to the lowest point I could get. I felt so lost. I felt nauseous every day. Each hour seemed like a day, each day seemed like a week. I wanted to hurry up and get the inevitable over with, even though I knew I needed some time to prepare myself emotionally.

I felt like I had disappointed my family and friends. They had been there with me through it all, from the original injury and for all of the surgeries that followed. They were always there to help me without ever being asked; they were my silent strength. I'm sure I never told any of them that, I just assumed they knew. I used to hate it when someone would comment to me on how wonderfully I had dealt with everything. They didn't have a clue. I was being strong on the outside for everybody else, but on the inside, I felt like I was slowly dying; this whole ordeal was sucking the life right out of me.

Yes, I had come a long way since the accident, but I certainly hadn't done it alone. I would never have made it this far by myself. I thought about my son—his 15th birthday was just around the corner. It reminded me of the day he turned 13, the big day a kid becomes a teenager, and we had to have his party in my hospital room. How shitty was that for a kid? I thought of all the times he had cooked, done laundry, or any other little thing I needed him to do. I thought of the previous year when I had developed an infection in the bone of my leg. I needed to have IV antibiotics daily for two months. I never would have even thought about asking him to help me with that, he was just a kid.

But one day, he volunteered; he asked me to show him how to take care of the IV itself and how to hook up the medicine that I required once a day. He knew it was hard for me and he wanted to help in any way that he could. I recalled the day I jokingly told him that I would need his help getting into the shower.

His response? "I'll help you get in there but I'm *NOT* staying!" But he really would have helped me if I'd needed him to. Although I was proud of him for being so helpful, I felt guilty that he had to deal with all of that. It's a lot of stress and worry for a child to have to carry.

I thought about my sisters and my best friend. It seems that one of them was always there to take me to a doctor appointment or the drug store or wherever I needed to go. I thought of the difficult times that I was never alone; one of them was always there for me; holding my hand, holding the puke bucket, or handing me a tissue to wipe my tears.

Sometimes just the mere presence of someone close can make the pain hurt a little less. I thought about my mother, and even now the thought of her being there through all of it brings tears to my eyes. I can't imagine what it must have been like for her. I probably seemed so helpless at times, and she just always knew. She never missed a surgery, even the unplanned ones that resulted from a quick doctor visit. I know for sure a person is never too old to need his or her mom. I can't imagine how difficult it must have been for her to see me like that. I was supposed to be a mother myself, but there were times when I just couldn't.

I remember sitting in Dr. Aslam's office discussing all of the technicalities of my impending amputation. I'm assuming that's what we were talking about, I don't really remember. I can see him vividly, his lips moving, but I can't tell you anything he may have said to me that day. He talked; I cried. I felt like I was never going to stop crying. Inside, I guess I never will. Dr. Aslam left me in the exam room for a minute while he went to summon a prosthetist who had an office in the same building. When they returned together a few moments later, I was still crying. I don't remember anything the prosthetist said, either.

The Unknowns of Amputation

The amputation was scheduled for April 11, 2001. An easy day for me to remember, it was my oldest brother's birthday. I wasn't afraid of having surgery; I had been through it so many times before. I knew all of the people who would be taking care of me, and I knew I would be in very capable hands. My primary fear was not knowing how much pain I would be in when I woke up. Surely, this would be far worse than any I had already been through, and I just didn't know what to expect. What I did know was that pain control would be the first priority when I woke up and I knew they wouldn't let me suffer. I did find some comfort in that.

Somewhere in the middle of all of this, my mother had been to see a new podiatrist in the area for an ongoing foot problem. He was young, only a couple of years older than me. Her problem would require minor surgery that he could do right in his office within a few days. She explained to him that I was having my leg amputated the following week so she didn't want to be laid up. She just didn't know how much I might need her help after my surgery. This led to an in-depth conversation between the two of them.

As a podiatrist, he was interested in hearing my story. I know that my mother broke down that day while she was talking to him. He comforted her immensely and he expressed an interest that he would like to meet me someday. My mother reported this visit with Dr. Smith to me later that day. She explained that he had just completed his schooling and opened a new office in Augusta in the three months before all of this was happening. She told me how welcoming he and his young wife were, and how the care and concern they showed her was overwhelmingly genuine. I was glad to know that my mother had gotten some comfort from them, this was not just a difficult time for me; it was a struggle for my whole family.

I called Dr. Smith myself the week before my amputation. Because he was fairly fresh out of school, I actually called him to see if he knew of any local educational programs for doctors that could benefit from the use of my amputated lower leg and foot. He made a couple of phone calls, but came up empty.

Through our phone conversations we decided I would stop at his office the following Tuesday after having all of my pre-op work done at the hospital, which was located a block from his office. Arriving at his office late in the morning, I brought my most recent x-rays for him to look at. Not because I wanted a second opinion and hoped he could save my leg, but because he had a special interest as a podiatrist. His wife greeted me at the reception desk. I told her my name and that I was there to speak with Dr. Smith.

He immediately appeared and had me follow him into his office. He closed the door and we both sat down. I wasn't there but just a few minutes when I was crying. It wasn't new, I cried every day at that point. But this time, I didn't even try to hold it back. I just let go and sobbed for what seemed like an eternity. I don't know what it was about him that was so reassuring, but it occurred to me as I sat there spilling my guts to a total stranger that this was an expression of grief I hadn't yet allowed myself to have, though it was totally normal for any patient in my shoes (pardon the pun).

He seemed so understanding and sympathetic, and it was the first time I had felt that it was okay for me to be real and honest about my anger and fear. I'm not sure how long I was there, but when I left, I felt more okay than I had when I got there. It wasn't because he made any thought-provoking or life-altering comments, he had just let me express what I was feeling and not make me feel stupid for being so emotional about it all. I was glad to have had the opportunity to make a new friend.

I had no idea that day how important Dr. Smith and his family would be in my recovery following the amputation. I don't remember much about the morning of my surgery. Everybody just seemed so somber. It was a sad day for all of us, not just me. My whole family was there that day and filled the entire waiting room. To my surprise, Dr. Smith and his wife had cleared their office calendar for the day and they both were there to wait with my family. I don't think I realized until that day how big of a deal this really was for them. They were grieving just as much as I was.

Saying Goodbyes

As they prepared to wheel me away to surgery, everyone needed a turn to give me one last hug and say goodbye. I wondered if this is what it felt like to be an inmate being led away for his lethal injection, because I was sure that, for the most part, my life was over. It's not like being whisked away for a Caesarean section where you know you'll have a precious little angel in the end. It's not like heading off for plastic surgery where you'll wake up with something new and improved. It was sad. It was a lot of pain and suffering, and still not ending up with anything good at the end.

When I gave the last hug and said the last goodbye, the stretcher moved and I began to cry. I didn't want my family to see me crying. I didn't want them to know how scared I was or how sad this whole thing felt. At that very moment, I didn't even care if I woke up after the surgery. Maybe that would be a good thing, I thought. I couldn't stand the thought of living a lifeless existence and I was sure that's what was in store for me. What amazes me the most is so many people who loved me came to be with me that day, but I had never felt more alone in my life.

Three-and-one-half weeks later, I found myself working for Dr. Smith, the podiatrist who had befriended my family and me at the time of my surgery. I could drive myself then, and was able to hobble into the office on my crutches. The plan was for me to get him caught up on all of his transcription and do some other light office duties until I got my prosthesis and was more mobile. Walking device-free in September, I was awarded the National Rehabilitation Services "Overcoming Barriers" award after Dr. Smith had nominated me.

Although I was quite mobile and walked with barely a limp, I wasn't able to spend as much time on my feet as I had hoped, and that interfered with my hopes for advancement from doing office work to being his full-time nurse. In late December, we amicably parted ways. Though I fully understood his need to replace me at that point, I was hugely disappointed at my body's lack of stamina and ability.

The physical recovery had been relatively easy. Six months after my amputation, I danced in a crowd and nobody knew I had the surgery. But I had grossly underestimated the emotional rollercoaster I found myself riding towards the end of that first year. I tried desperately to figure out where I belonged in life. Now with no job, and more than likely no nursing career, alcohol became a means to escape depressing thoughts.

A New Outlook

In April, just one year after having my leg amputated, I took a job at my local hospital's anti-coagulation clinic. It was a lesser job than what I was trained to do, but it was *something* and, for my mental health, I really needed to be working. I worked at the clinic for just more than two years and discovered therapy and healing through writing.

With a new purpose, I had to write my story to help all of the other people with amputations out there who struggled like I had. I wanted to let them know that amputation is not necessarily a bad thing. If the limb you have is making you sick and causing you pain, where is the quality in life? I also knew I had a good "in" with healthcare providers who try to be emotionally supportive to our new amputee patients, but aren't really aware of the hurdles we face.

In 2008, I took a job as a dialysis nurse at my local hospital. I never thought I would get more out of that job than what I put in, but we have many amputee patients and I was able to bond with them in a very special way. I don't hesitate to share my story with them. It's important for them to see that life goes on despite misfortune. I can't work a 10-hour shift like everybody else does, but I can keep up with them while I am there.

I became a certified amputee peer visitor, and speak to people about my journey whenever the opportunity arises. I am a much better nurse than I ever was before. The most valuable lesson I have learned is that tough times don't last, but tough people do.

Building Resilience

Time is a great healer

Get back to work

Write

Share your journey

Reach out to others with a similar disability

Life goes on

Carolyn McKinzie lives in Randolph, ME, and works as a dialysis nurse at Maine Medical Center. Carolyn went to nursing school at Kennebec Valley Community College.

She is a member of Hanger Prosthetic's "Amputee Empowerment Program" and serves as a certified peer counselor and regional coordinator for Amputee Empowerment Partners for the Portland, Maine area. Carolyn also wrote a soon to be published book about the experience called, 'Walk softly: A woman's journey through limb loss." *She is a blog contributor for "Abled Amputees of America"* http://www.abledamputees.org/#!heart-of-inspiration/csv7. *She can be reached at* blueeyedlady1101@yahoo.com.

Suggested Reading

McKinzie, C. (2012). Recovery and Reunion. A mother and daughter's reflections on the long journey back. *InMotion, 22*(1), 30-31. Retrieved on October 20, 2013 from: http://www.amputee-coalition.org/inmotion_online/inmotion-22-01-web/pubData/source/jan-feb_2012fb.pdf

COMMENTARY

By Leslie Pitt Schneider, JD, RN, CCRC(ACRP), HT(ASCP)

Though her own experience, Carolyn candidly recounts her personal journey in coping with limb loss. In her career as a licensed practical nurse, she was trained to be "emotionally supportive" to those coping with limb loss. Now, with the fate of life, she reverses roles and becomes the patient. She vividly recounts the pain and struggles that she endured, prior, during, and after her limb loss. From the initial accident, through the countless conservation surgeries to the ultimate amputation of her leg, this chapter describes the feelings that healthcare professionals rarely experience themselves. Carolyn guides the reader through her emotional pain of losing a limb to her realization that, despite it all, "tough times don't last, but tough people do."

In addition to resources relative to their individual rights under the ADA, nurses experiencing life with limb loss may benefit from involvement in peer networks, or support groups. Through its Peer Support Network, the Amputee Coalition coordinates peer visits between people requesting such services and their peer-visitor-trained volunteers, who are also people coping with limb loss. Likewise, the Amputee Coalition maintains an active database of nearly 300 peer networks and support groups throughout the United States, in addition to several other countries. Finally, the Peer Support Network provides articles, websites, and other information relative to limb loss.

Leslie Pitt Schneider, JD, RN, CCRC(ACRP), HT(ASCP) is a nurse and an attorney. She is the clinical & regulatory affairs, manager, legal compliance Otto Bock Healthcare and a board member of the Amputee Coalition. Leslie has had a lower limb amputation for the last 38 years of her life after losing her leg when she was run over by a gravel truck at the age of six. She practiced as a nurse for many years before attending law school. Leslie can be reached at Leslie.Schneider@ottobock.com .

Suggested Reading

Amputee Coalition: http://www.amputee-coalition.org/index.html

Disability.gov: https://www.disability.gov

EEOC: http://www.eeoc.gov/policy/docs/accommodation.html

Peer Support Network: http://www.amputee-coalition.org/npn_about.html

14 WEAVE YOUR SKILLS IN WITH YOUR CHALLENGE: NURSING WITH LOW VISION

By Susan Nordemo, RN, CH, Reiki Master Teacher

On March 6, 1945, I was born in Cambridge, MA. My mother saw my eye defects before the doctor saw them. What it was called back then I am not sure, but now it is known as coloboma—which comes from the Greek word meaning "curtailed." The word is used to describe conditions where normal tissue in or around the eye is missing from birth. My pupils were affected, back to the retinas. I have no vision at the top of both eyes. If I had been born with this defect over the macula, I would have been totally blind. So, from birth I was blessed with good fortune.

Since graduating from Beverly Hospital School of Nursing in Boston in 1965, I have worked full time at many different jobs, owned a temporary nursing agency, and now have my own business that I started in 1998 providing hypnosis, Reiki, and Emotional Freedom Technique. Trying to make a "go" of my business at the beginning, I moved from Massachusetts to New Hampshire and didn't work in nursing for a while.

Until 2000, I had good corrected vision in both eyes. Then I was diagnosed with cataracts as a result of 30 years of smoking. *Yes*, smoking can cause cataracts—back then I was never warned and even stopping smoking 15 years earlier and it didn't help— the damage was already done.

Later on, when I decided to return to nursing, my vision had dramatically changed. When I went for an interview at a nursing home, I recognized "trouble" when I could not see the application well enough to complete it. I went home and went into a depression, not wanting to see or speak to any of my friends. At this point, I had no passion for my business. I soon realized I had a choice— I could stay depressed or get help. I realized when you make the choice to take control and take action, the fear drops away. Fear is a result of inaction.

Getting Proactive

A call to my state department of low vision (services for the blind and visually impaired) resulted in a visit the next morning and delivery of a free zoom text program for my computer and large labels for my keyboard. A job coach came to the house the next day. As luck would have it, just before she arrived, a flyer showed up in the mail with information about a company looking for night nurses to do telephone triage. I thought this sounded perfect! When you take action, the universe provides everything that you need to succeed. You only have to learn how to recognize it.

The coach helped me rework my resume. She prepared everything for me, coached me on how to handle the interview, and drove me to the agency. The next day I had the job. After accepting the position, I told the agency that I had low vision and the state department of low vision would be providing all the necessary tools to assist me free of charge. I have been there more than four years and love the job.

My business is also thriving and I am always looking at new avenues to apply my skills using hypnosis and Emotional Freedom Technique (EFT). Many of my sessions can be done over the telephone so in the event that I can no longer do nursing triage, I will have a good income.

When I was diagnosed as legally blind, which I waited to do because I was in denial, I consequently found out that in Nashua, NH, when you are legally blind you can get half of your property tax taken off and a FREE FISHING LICENSE! So for two weeks I was walking around the house saying "You know GOD I would rather pay my full property tax and get my vision back"…. Besides I don't like to fish.

Nurses with disabilities should consider holistic nursing because of the various career opportunities. A nurse with low vision or hearing loss can be a hypnotist or Reiki Master. Our intentions as caregivers can be very strong and so enhanced when we take the holistic approach. Visit the web site of The American Holistic Nurses Association for more information: http://www.ahna.org.

For those of you who are already nurses, you need to know that you have an incredible set of skills that can be applied many different ways. It is like a tapestry where you weave your skills in with your challenge to produce a work of art.

For those of you who are considering nursing and have been told it cannot be done, find a different way, create a new way and never take "no" for an answer unless it is your decision. All no means is next opportunity (N.O.)! Ask for help from people who will encourage you every step of the way. Be only in the presence of those who are a positive influence. Einstein said, "Matter is energy."

A dear friend and mentor of mine says, "It's energy that matters." If you think it, you can create it.

Building Resilience

Take action

Be creative

Surround yourself with positive influences

Don't take "no" for an answer

Start your own business

Susan Nordemo lives in New Hampshire. Her business is called Monarch Healthcoaching http://www.monarchhealthcoaching.com. *She continues to do telephone triage with Ali Care Medical Management. Susan can be reached at* sue@monarchhealthcoaching.com.

Suggested Reading

The American Holistic Nurses Association: http://www.ahna.org/

International Association of Reiki Professionals:http://www.iarp.org/

COMMENTARY

By Detra Bannister, RN

Susan's story is similar to my own in that immediately after my vision loss, I was distressed and in an overwhelming quandary about what to do. How would I continue working? What questions do I need to ask? On whom do I call to get answers? Will anyone encourage me, believe in me, or support me? Where does one find help in this situation? Is there any such thing as a successfully employed nurse with vision loss??

After all, the solution for a nurse with vision loss is composed of many interconnected parts and, even with help, figuring this all out can be an overwhelming process. I was thrilled with the points of building resilience and from experience, know that they are spot on. As I read them, even 18 years after winning this battle, my heart was lifted and encouraged.

For nurses who have lost sight, first of all, let me encourage you that this is not the end of the world. Give yourself permission to grieve if you have lost a significant amount of vision. I made the mistake of not grieving because I was so occupied with all of the practical aspects of survival such as keeping my job, home, finding transportation, paying bills, etc. Years later, it caught up with me in a big way. Learn from my mistake and don't indulge in endless grief any more than you would ignore it. Nurse your loss by getting up and getting help. Yes, I know that asking for help is a hard thing for nurses to do because that is what WE do: provide help.

Get Help from Agencies

The best way to get this help is to get in touch with a state, local, or private rehabilitation agency for the blind or visually impaired. They are equipped to help you in all aspects of putting life back together.

For the most part, nursing is a very visual profession but it is also very knowledge based. By virtue of this fact, once blindness compensatory skills have been mastered, we can custom design and use systems for storing knowledge, facts, and rules about the work we do. Therefore, we can still represent the world of nursing in a unique and professional manner.

Furthermore, we have the added bonus of compassion and deeper insight based on our own struggles with disability.

When representing yourself to a perspective employer, the best thing you can do is to be at ease and comfortable in your skin as a person with a disability. If you know you have the skills and ability to perform the task of a given job talk about how you would perform those tasks. You might take one or two of your high- or low-tech devices that enable you to do everyday tasks such as a lighted magnifier, braille, or voice note taker or hand-held memo recorder. You could present pictures and information about talking blood pressure machines, scales, thermometers, or computer software to put the employer's mind at ease, and help them understand how easily and inexpensively accommodations can be made.

The more comfortable you are with yourself and the more you understand about the accommodations you need to do your job, the better you can make a potential employer comfortable with your disability while, at the same time, helping them understand your many transferable skills, and abilities.

Career Connections

The career education and exploration program of the American Foundation for the Blind, AFB CareerConnect®, can be a tremendous help to someone looking to go back to work in a specific field after vision loss. This program is free and has specific information for job seekers and employers. Reading the articles in these two sections and using the interactive components of this program will help you understand what employers are thinking, what they need to know, and how best to interact with them. You will also learn ways of finding work, doing successful job interviews, when to disclose your disability, getting hired, keeping your job, climbing the ladder at work, and more.

Perhaps the most valuable ingredient that AFB CareerConnect adds to the process of re-entering the workforce is the mentoring component. Over 1,000 successfully employed individuals with varying degrees of vision loss that range from considerable useful vision to no useful vision, volunteer to mentor others in their career paths. These people work in more than 300 occupational fields in today's labor market and, yes, there are nurses, doctors, occupational therapists, medical transcriptionists, pharmacists, and more. To engage a mentor and learn more about this program go to www.afb.org/careerconnect.

Detra Bannister, RN, has worked as a surgical, community, and school health nurse. She works as a CareerConnect Program Specialist for the American Foundation for the Blind. She can be reached at careerconnect@afb.net.

15 LOVING OURSELVES EXACTLY AS WE ARE: NURSING AFTER A STROKE

By Connie Stallone Adleman, RN

When we love ourselves exactly as we are, we begin to become better able to transform how we think about ourselves and how others think about us. This is when our inner healing starts to take place. Loving ourselves in spite of our disabilities is empowering. Loving myself is how I put my disabilities into perspective after I had a stroke and ultimately was able to feel whole and complete again. Distinct forces in my life helped me to go on to have a remarkable recovery and return to teaching.

I was a nurse.

I had practiced psychiatric nursing for 37 years and I had studied spirituality for 20 years. My husband of 26 years, an actor and a playwright, who stayed as far away from the healthcare system as he could, seemed to know instinctively what I needed from the moment the stroke began and all through my recovery.

What happened to me??

In August of 1996 on a day filled with sunshine in New York City, I didn't feel well, but I kept telling myself it was nothing serious. It was Saturday and I was scheduled to fill in for another nursing instructor whose father was having surgery that morning. I also didn't want to break the unwritten rule in nursing— *nurses don't call in sick on weekends.*

Within an hour or so of lecturing, I started to feel light-headed and somewhat spacey; yet I continued to teach and ignored what was happening to me. In the middle of the lecture, I walked over to the chalkboard and I began writing my name in various ways. When I decided to sit down in the chair behind the desk, my depth perception was off, and I could not determine how far I had to go in order to sit. Still standing, I picked the test papers up off the desk and not only dropped them, but then, I could not figure out how to pick them up. Feeling frightened and at the same time wanting to protect my students, I decided to leave the classroom to talk with the other nursing instructor at the school that day.

Outside in the hallway, I felt as though every thought I had was moving in slow motion while my fear was moving in accelerated waves. Holding onto either side of the wall along the corridor until I reached the other classroom, I felt some relief when I finally saw the other nursing instructor. I weakly waved to her and to her students and continued to slowly move towards the teacher's lounge with my colleague right behind me. "I think I may be having a stroke," I said, bursting into tears.

And after haltingly telling her what had just happened and after she did a quick assessment, she touched my arm and sadly said, "I think you may be right, and you need to get to the hospital immediately."

Within minutes, I was on my way to the emergency room, which quickly became an anxiety-provoking maze of decisions that soon turned utterly frightening. Especially when my husband, Darrel, and I disagreed with the neurology consultant who wanted to attempt a procedure— that would only give me a 50-50 chance of survival. Darrel and I chose what we felt would be a less invasive approach and I was admitted into the hospital. The next morning, I woke up to find that I had left-sided paralysis, slurred speech, and my thoughts were slowed down as well.

My life as I had known it seemed to be over. I wanted to dissolve. I felt as though I had lost everything. I began to blame myself, feeling guilty about being overweight and having high blood pressure, for years. I had tried everything to get these two issues under control. Most of my life they had remained a constant source of turmoil for me. I silently screamed at all of the stress I had been carrying around with me. It was at this moment that all of the tears that had been stuck in my heart and in my throat since the classroom episode erupted into guttural sounds.

A nurse came into my room and after quickly checking my IV, held my hand and said, "Just let go. Just keep letting that go." And I knew that in that moment that out of all of the people that I had been surrounded with for the past 24 hours, it was only my husband, and now this nurse who knew exactly what I was feeling.

Soon after, my brother-in-law, who is a spiritual practitioner, called me from California. "You have to believe that your left arm and leg are moving, and that your speech and your thoughts are clear," he said. "Hold onto that vision. Meditate on it. And give thanks for your life."

I had been studying spirituality for a few years by then and I did meditate regularly; however, I wasn't sure how much I believed that his suggestion could help me in terms of a stroke. I was a nurse after all and grounded in facts and reality. Plus, I was having difficulty concentrating on anything other than my grief. My thoughts were so fragmented that I couldn't really relax enough to begin to meditate. I tried to focus on the IV bottle by counting the drips. I listened to the familiar sounds of the hospital going on outside my door and I began to pray.

Why Me?

Suddenly, I thought, this is not fair. I wanted my brownie points that must have accumulated over the 37 years that I had practiced and taught psychiatric nursing, and had helped so many people. I had met everyone's needs and had given so much of myself. How could this be happening to me? I heard a three-year-old voice inside of me, crying, "Not fair!" And then I also heard my adult nurse voice saying, "You're going to have to face this." *How?* I wondered as my tears flowed.

"I spoke to Scott and I agree with him," my husband said later that morning. "Let your doctor take care of your medical treatments and we'll take care of your inner healing."

"How could I possibly do that?" I cried. "How can I overcome the damage that's been done and might continue? How can I possibly recover from a stroke?"

"You can start by relaxing," he said. "Take a few deep breaths and keep affirming that, "on the invisible, you are in the process of recovering. Let that be your supportive thought."

"I'll never be the same," I said.

"Connie, you may be different from now on. You may have some disabilities, but you are still *whole* within yourself."

I cried a lot that day and for many days after. However, I did keep going "within" through meditation. I also kept connecting with that invisible part of me that I agreed could help me to heal from the emotional pain that I was feeling.

Hard Work in Therapy

Soon, my days were filled with physical, occupational, and speech therapy sessions. My days were enhanced by numerous talks with the nursing staff. "It's as though the nurses have formed a wagon train around you," Darrel said. Together, my husband and I also integrated the following healing techniques into my daily routine:

Deep breathing and relaxation techniques in order to lower my stress level.

Affirmations such as, *my left arm and my left leg are moving* and *my thoughts and speech are clear*— to help me with my self-image.

From my studies of Louise Hay's work, author of, *You Can Heal Your Life* (1987), I knew that positive affirmations were powerful and would help me to implant more positive thoughts into my mind. I also began to forgive myself for having a stroke and for not taking better care of myself. Once I began the process of forgiving myself, I found that it was not easy and that it initially conjured up feelings of resentment and anxiety. The more I practiced though, the more easily I began to love myself. And as soon as I begin to accept myself exactly as I was, I started on my road to recovery.

When my husband and I moved to California in the 1980s, the New Age Movement was just beginning. I began to attend workshops led by Louise L. Hay. Her teachings helped me to learn the value of using positive affirmations and loving myself more. Prior to having a stroke, reading her book made me feel safe. Yet, even though I had appreciated all of this knowledge, I had disabled myself by continuing to put everything and everyone first as I continued my workaholic behavior, and had taken little time out for me. Like many nurses, I had been conditioned to believe that patients' needs were first. As a result, I often neglected my own and my medical issues began to catch up with me. My weight and blood pressure were now out of control and I was constantly exhausted.

A New Perspective

And I had not yet learned that in order to have the life that I desired, I would have to change my negative thoughts to more positive ones. I would have to begin to love myself enough to begin to put my needs first. This was not an easy task after practicing nursing for more than 30 years and being the quintessential caregiver.

In spite of my fear at the beginning, I knew that I would have to take a proactive stance if I wanted to recover. I would have to use my nursing expertise and savvy, and apply it myself. I had to let go of my limiting beliefs and realize that I was more than my disabilities. I had to remember who I was and who I had been. As a nurse, I knew how patients healed and I knew how patients limited their own progress. Blame and guilt did not help you to recover. I knew how valuable expressing my thoughts and feelings would be. And I knew that I had to stay fully present in my care plan and not live in the past or the future. There was only *now*. I had to take it one step at a time and one day at a time. And, most of all, I would have to love myself and love every part of me, including the disabled parts.

I turned within. I began to use affirmations that could help me to improve the quality of my life and in particular, the state of my recovery. Two of my daily affirmations were: *I love myself exactly as I am.* And *I love taking care of me now and being taken care of.* I also used gratitude to help me cope by affirming; *I give thanks to all the parts of myself.* And *I give thanks for my life.*

I had practiced psychiatric nursing since 1960. I found through my career that the longer I had practiced psychiatric nursing, the more I had discovered the relationship between the mind and body and its impact on illness. I therapeutically applied my knowledge to my patients, but learned that I had not applied it enough to myself.

The Power of Writing

Then something happened that would empower me and put me on the road to recovery. My husband gave me a notebook and said, "I think it's really important for you to journal this experience."

"I can hardly function," I said. "How can I possibly write?"

"You can cry all you want to," he said. "But you still have to get involved in your rehabilitation. You love to write. Your career is all about expressing your feelings. You taught your patients to express theirs and now writing will give you that opportunity."

"What should I write?"

"Hon, you know what to do. Write down your thoughts," my husband said.

Suddenly that practical, down-to-earth, New York nurse who was highly skilled at handling emergencies, who was an expert in crisis intervention, and who was exceptional at motivating patients was behaving like a frightened child.

"You have to follow the principles you've been reading, studying, and teaching," my husband said. "Along with meditating and doing guided imagery, you can also write. I would go beyond the limits of this stroke now."

"My left hand is paralyzed." I said.

"Hon, you're right-handed."

I finally agreed that along with fully participating in my medical, nursing, and rehabilitation plan, I would begin to use my journal as a therapeutic experience. Dr. James Pennebaker, a psychologist, conducted studies that proved that writing during an illness or in response to a physical or emotional issue was not only therapeutic, but also a way to help people physically get better (Pennebaker, 1997, 2004).

Writing helped me to deal with my initial disabilities. And it helped me to articulate my vision for my recovery. My journals have been turned into a book, *A Bold Stroke: Healing from Within* that is nearing completion. I have also written a continuing education course for www.ExceptionalNurse.com titled *Writing Your Way to Health & Healing: An Interactive Workshop* (2013*),* along with an article titled, "A holistic approach to rehab,*"* for the Stroke Association's Magazine (2006).

A nursing colleague gave me a Louise Hay tape, titled, *Self-Healing: Creating Health* (1988). Each night I listened to that tape. And even though I would fall asleep throughout most of it, the next day, I would remember phrases from that tape such as, *"guilt and blame are useless emotions."* Another morning, I recalled that she had said, *"Approve of and accept yourself exactly as you are."*

Peaceful Visualization

Darrel also often led me through the healing technique, "Creative Visualization" written by the metaphysical author, Shakti Gawain (2002). After encouraging me to do a relaxation technique, my husband would encourage me to visualize that I was in a peaceful state. And that I was functioning perfectly. For example, he would say, *"Imagine that you are speaking normally, walking easily again, and thinking clearly."*

And in order for me to learn how to speak clearly again, my husband began to supplement my daily sessions with my speech therapist by coaching me each evening. As an actor and a playwright, he had studied speech and he had a great deal of information regarding pronunciation and articulation. One evening during a Creative Visualization technique exercise, my husband added, *"Relax and think about speaking clearly. Imagine you've even lost your Bronx accent."* Both of us knew that that was never going to happen!

The scene had been set. My choice had been made. I would participate full on in my medical and rehabilitation plan and I would integrate inner healing techniques into my daily routine. And Darrel and I would work on this together. It would be a turning point in my illness. For however disabled I was, I was still alive. "You have to become your own best nurse now," my husband said. So, I opened my journal and I wrote a SOAP note about myself.

S- Patient says she wants to recover.

O-Patient is doing nothing tangible in that direction except crying.

A-Patient needs to actively practice holistic and spiritual techniques on a daily basis.

P- Help patient put on her earphones twice a day to listen to healing tapes. Give her a pen and her journal each day and encourage her to write.

Forgiveness was the next hurdle I had to overcome. To forgive myself for being so overweight, having high blood pressure, and putting everyone else's needs in front of mine was not easy to do. I wrote, "*I forgive myself for any of my doubts that I have about my health. I forgive and love myself now.*" And, I also wrote, "*I forgive myself for not paying more attention to me and to my healthcare needs.*"

Meditating each morning while listening to Louise Hay's tape and using creative meditation helped me to greatly lower my stress level and blood pressure. I also began practicing a relaxation technique that helped me to achieve a greater sense of emotional well-being and I looked forward to my subsequent sessions.

During one of my first outpatient rehabilitation experiences, the occupational therapist asked me to demonstrate the hand-washing technique that is part of our daily routine as health professionals. When I found that I couldn't remember the sequence and kept taking paper towels out of the dispenser to stall for time, my heart started beating rapidly, my mouth became dry, I felt like crying, and I knew from the pressure in my head, that my blood pressure was rising.

Deep Breathing to Refocus

And then, the therapist said the magic words. "Take three slow deep breaths and relax." By doing that I was able to refocus my thoughts, especially as I affirmed, "I easily remember the steps to washing my hands." I felt less threatened and I finally accomplished the task. She helped me to lower my anxiety, focus on the task and remember the steps. Stress management is a truly effective tool before an occupational therapy session.

Learning how to walk again was another challenge. I ended up having some long-term physical therapy and using water therapy as part of my treatment program. I had to keep turning my fear into a challenge to succeed.

About two years after having a stroke, my husband and I moved to Seneca Falls in Central New York and began living in a cottage by a lake, which really moved my recovery along because it was so peaceful. Soon, my speech was clearer, my thinking was back to normal, and I had no visible signs of having had a stroke. And one sunny day, I gave up the last cane that I would ever use while walking. I was ready to go back to work.

I met with Eileen Gage, RN, vice president of nursing at Finger Lakes Health in Geneva, NY. She hired me to teach a four-day program for her in-service education department. After that, I created classes on stress management and empowerment that I taught to her nursing staff for the next several years.

When I later asked her why she had hired a nurse with a disability, she wrote:

"In my 30-year career as a clinician and administrator, I have found that exceptional nurses are individuals who seek to understand the caring experience from the patient's perspective. Nurses who master this skill have a dramatic impact on the lives they touch. Nurses who have accepted the challenge created by a disability and continue to pursue their passion, often have a greater capacity to understand the experience, establish the therapeutic relationship and convey to other nurses the type of support and encouragement required to achieve a health goal. They bring a unique and beneficial perspective to their chosen nursing role. I met Connie in 1999, and was impressed with her passion to help others succeed, to develop confidence and power through positive thinking. Her psychiatric nursing experience, advocacy work, teaching and group dynamics programs clearly evidenced her knowledge on the subject of personal development.

However, it was her story of recovery from stroke that enabled me to see her teaching and philosophy in action."

The stroke was over. My new life had begun. And I gave thanks for arriving at this point. Along with completing my book and teaching, I now also offer a six-week holistic, motivational coaching program for individual nurses, healthcare agencies, and organizations. As part of that coaching program, I offer clients a safe place to express their feelings, make positive changes in their life, and learn how to love themselves exactly as they are.

Building Resilience

Love yourself exactly as you are

Writing can help you heal

Use creative visualizations

Give thanks

Connie Stallone Adleman, RN, is a stroke survivor and lives in New York. She is a nurse educator, author, speaker, and coach. She can be reached at dcwriter2005@yahoo.com.

References

Adleman, C. (2006, May/June) A holistic approach to rehabilitation. *Stroke Connection Magazine*, http://www.strokeassociation.org/idc/groups/stroke-public/@wcm/@hcm/@sta/documents/downloadable/ucm_314586.pdf

Adleman, C. (2006). Writing your way to health and healing, Retrieved on March 15, 2013 at http://exceptionalnurse.com/pdf/ONLINEWORKSHOPFORNURSES.pdf

Gawain, S. (2002) *Creative visualization*, New World Library, Novato, CA

Hay, L.L. (1987). *You can heal your life*, Hay House, Carlsbad, CA

Hay, L. L. (1988) *Self-healing: Creating health*, [CD/audiobook]. Carlsbad, CA: Hay House

Pennebaker, J. W. (2004*). Writing to heal: A guided journal for recovering from trauma and emotional upheaval.* Oakland, CA: New Harbinger Press.

Pennebaker, J. W. (1997). *Opening up: The healing power of expressing emotions.* New York: Guilford Press.

COMMENTARY

By Tommye-Karen Mayer, BA

How honestly, vividly, and bravely Connie relates the long emotional stages to surviving a stroke. Every stroke survivor needs to know we've all been devastated and been thorough our own "not-so-inspirational reactions to our new reality." I'm chuckling as I write this. Connie so carefully relates her path to recruiting the knowledge she had and acquiring what she needed to accomplish in her recovery to the new her: post-stroke.

What a mental sea change it is to traverse from caregiver to care-receiver—all that you've patiently given to others, you now must give yourself and receive from others. Not only has half your body mutinied and ceased responding to instruction from your brain, but your world's upside-down: You're getting care, not giving it.

Connie also demonstrates the importance of the taking time to heal and relearn how to accomplish routine activities of daily living. The ability to manage your own needs will increase your independence and confidence. This will be beneficial if a return to work is your goal.

In thinking about advising a stroke-surviving nurse or a nurse with upper extremity limb loss intent upon returning to work, I would suggest she or he think about the tasks involved every day. While I am not a nurse, I certainly have seen nurses at work many times and in many settings. Nurses work in different roles. Knowing exactly what it is you want to do is key to figuring out how to do what you want. What is involved in the nursing position you want? Of course, there won't simply be a single "it" and some of the "its" may involve multi-step processes you'll want to examine in light of your one-handedness or other limitation.

In writing my book, *One-Handed in a Two-Handed World*, I identified keys to managing single-handedness, which I call "The Three Secrets." These secrets are: four fingers and a thumb (recognizing you don't have one hand, but five independent digits); body positioning (organizing the rest of you to help leverage your project); and gadgets (assistive devices to help you accomplish your specific task; Mayer, 2013). With practice, these Three

Secrets will help you accomplish your tasks after you've clearly identified for yourself precisely what you want to do.

Explore medical equipment made for use with one hand (e.g. one-hand manual blood pressure cuffs, one-hand adjustable IV poles, and one-hand syringes). Explore the nursing literature for information about doing procedures such as donning sterile gloves with one hand (Maheady & Fleming, 2005; Fleming & Maheady, 2008; Maheady & Fleming, 2012). This will increase your confidence and help you answer the questions related to "How will you be able to do_____?"

It is also very important to organize your workspace to work for you (Mayer, 2013). Those four fingers and thumb can't be wasted by just holding. They need to be free to do things.

Inspiring Others

After you've carefully considered all the tasks involved in the nursing position you want, and thought through the one-handed work-arounds, you'll have the confidence to assure the hiring manager. You will also be bringing valuable experience to your nursing job. Not only have you experienced first-hand what patients go through, you continue to experience the challenges of having a disability. Imagine what a boost it would have been to your recovery if you had seen an effectively functioning stroke survivor or upper extremity amputee nurse when you were trying to figure out how you could ever manage without that other hand.

Your experience can be a powerful value-add that none of the other applicants will have. Take advantage of that experience with the confidence you gained from problem-solving the work in light of getting it all done with what you do have; that so much of you that still functions, and functions more effectively because you've become more aware. I often laugh over how wasteful of their resources two-handed people can be.

Tommye-Karen Mayer, BA has been a stroke survivor since June 1981 when she survived a cerebral hemorrhage pursuant to an arteriovenous malformation (AVM) at 23 years of age. She is the author of One-Handed in a Two-Handed World *and* Teaching Me to Run.

References

Fleming. S. & Maheady, D. (2008). *Nursing with the hand you are given: A message of hope for nursing students with disabilities.* [DVD] Spokane: Washington State University Intercollegiate College of Nursing.

Maheady, D.C. & Fleming, S. (2005, Summer). Nursing with the hand you are given. *Minority Nurse*, 50-54. http://www.exceptionalnurse.com/DegreesofSuccess.pdf

Maheady, D. & Fleming, S. (2012). Missing a limb, but not a heart. *Reflections on Nursing Leadership*, 38 (1). Retrieved online March 25, 2012 at http://www.reflectionsonnursingleadership.org/Pages/Vol38_1_Maheady_Fleming.aspx

Mayer, T. K. (2013). *One–handed in a two-handed world.* (4th ed.) New York: DiaMedica Publishing.

16 FUTURE PLANNING

By Donna Carol Maheady, ARNP, EdD

Imagine that you become disabled from an accident, stroke, or illness. After rehabilitation, you long to return to nursing—to the work you love. Questions may arise, such as: Will my position still be there? Will accommodations be made for me, if necessary? The answer is sometimes "yes" and sometimes "no." The opportunity to work as a nurse in your previous position may not be available, no matter how much experience or commitment you have.

Realistically, most nurses won't work as staff nurses on medical-surgical floors for 40 years. Planning for the future should begin today. Everyone needs to explore the "What if?" questions about themselves, their family, career, and finances in order to formulate a plan of action should disability happen or an existing disability exacerbates.

Often, nurses are so busy caring for others that they forget about caring for themselves. Nurses should consider doing a yearly inventory or career checkup based on age, personal, and family health status, finances, and professional and healthcare industry trends. As a way to remember, this annual checkup could be scheduled at the start of a new year or on a birthday or anniversary. Notes could be kept in a journal. Answers to the following questions will help to formulate a personal/professional care plan:

What if I get sick or become disabled?

What if my disability exacerbates or is disclosed?

What if I'm in an accident?

What if I hurt my back at work?

What if a patient hits me?

Can I be a staff nurse for my entire nursing career?

What if my position is eliminated or my hospital closes?

Do I have enough in savings to retire?

What if my parent, spouse, or child gets sick?

In addition to a yearly professional checkup, nurses need to stay as healthy as possible, take care of themselves, and continue learning new skills throughout their careers. Whenever possible, go back to school for an advanced degree; volunteer to be a school nurse on your day off; give flu shots at flu shot clinic; work as a camp nurse; go on a medical mission trip; or sign up with an agency and do an occasional home visit. Learn medical coding or transcription. Teach a class. Become a CPR or yoga instructor. Follow your heart and interests, but above all have a Plan B.

Additional suggestions to facilitate resilience include the following:

- Get regular medical checkups.

- Eat healthy, exercise, laugh, play, and give thanks.

- Don't drink in excess or smoke.

- Recognize when you may be burned out. These times should serve as a wake-up call to first take care of yourself so you can be of service to others.

- Reduce stress. Try yoga or a dance class. Learn a new craft or hobby, such as knitting or scrapbook making. Take a cooking class or guitar lessons.

- Recognize your limitations. Be honest with yourself and others. Say "no" when appropriate.

- Ask yourself the tough questions: Can I perform the essential skills of the job with or without accommodations? Conduct an inventory of your strengths and weaknesses. Compare this list with the essential skills or technical standards of the nursing position you have or are considering.

• Be prepared to answer questions, such as, "How will you perform CPR? How will you lift, transfer, and ambulate a patient? How will you hear a patient's call bell or the telephone?" Identify any areas of possible concern.

• Address any issues head on, with patient safety foremost in mind. Address potential concerns your employers may have by demonstrating or describing how you would meet technical standards with or without reasonable accommodations.

• Consider whether to disclose carefully. Your need to disclose your disability to your employer is proportional to your need for accommodations. It's like wearing glasses or contacts: If your vision aid sufficiently corrects your vision, then you don't need to talk about it with your employer. If you can fulfill your duties with your aids, don't make a big deal of it. If you need to use a wheelchair, scooter, or sign language interpreter, your employer will need to know.

• Do your homework. It is your responsibility to do the research and know what accommodations to ask for. Your employer isn't responsible for knowing what you need. If accommodations are provided, be prepared to answer questions and deal proactively with ignorant comments or biased behavior.

• Seek assistance from attorneys, advocacy organizations, union officers, and other nurses with disabilities if you need to make a case for being allowed to continue practicing as a nurse. Cherish your nursing license. Don't give it up! You worked hard for it and it can be very difficult to reactivate.

• Study the laws that offer protection to employees with disabilities, such as the American with Disabilities Act of 1990 and amendments in 2008, and the Family and Medical Leave Act of 1993.

• Familiarize yourself with the regulations and services provided by the Bureau of Workers' Compensation and your state's vocational rehabilitation agency. If you become a recipient of services from workers' compensation or vocational rehabilitation, learn all you can about the agency and services offered. There may be an employment opportunity for you within the system designed to help you.

• Visit the website of your state's nursing board. Review your state's Nurse Practice Act. Research whether or not your state has practice restrictions or a limited license for nurses with disabilities.

• Volunteer in a nursing home or school. For example, Robin Mazzuca, RN, MPH, has multiple sclerosis. She and her service dog, Georgia, volunteer at nursing homes, schools, and rehabilitation facilities. Volunteer to be the nurse at your local Walk for the Cure. Teach a class for newly diagnosed people with your disability or lead a support group. Volunteer with the Red Cross Condolence program (Lynch, 2013). Volunteer opportunities can be an opportunity to learn new skills and gain experience. Often, the experience can lead to an employment opportunity.

• Be a change agent. Examine the mission and value statements of your place of employment. Is dedication to employees a value? Is health promotion, safe working conditions, support, respect, loyalty, diversity, flexibility, and equal opportunity included? If not, work to make changes. Study your hospital's or employer's policies for employees. What provisions are made for nurses to return to work on a light-duty assignment? Volunteer to work on a committee to develop strategies for accommodating nurses who need temporary or permanent accommodations.

• Network. Professional contacts are vital in planning for the future. When you attend meetings, conferences, or continuing education programs, sit with new people and introduce yourself. Collect business cards, names, numbers, and e-mail addresses. Reconnect with old friends on Facebook. Follow up with new contacts, and stay in touch. Friendships and successful ventures can be built by sharing ideas, resources, and leads. If you become a good networker, you also become a good listener, conversationalist, and resource for others — even if you're the one looking for the leads.

• Join professional organizations. Join your state's nursing association or organizations related to your disability. Attend meetings and serve on committees. Run for office. The experience and the networking opportunities will benefit you in the future.

• Learn new skills. Stay current with computer skills and the latest technology. If an inservice is offered about new equipment, try to attend. Study a foreign language or take a sign language or lip reading course.

• Continue your education. Consider working on your AD, BSN, MS, or doctoral degree. Go back to school with a friend. Having a friend in the same situation can help you overcome any rough spots. Take it slowly if you need to. Consider a minor in a subject that may open other doors e.g., counseling, social work, disability studies, business, psychology, nutrition, fitness/wellness, nursing informatics, rural/border/global/international health, or a foreign language. Obtain and maintain certifications in your specialty area.

• Heal yourself and others. Consider becoming a holistic nurse. Learn to integrate complementary and alternative modalities (CAM) into clinical practice to treat the whole person. Examples include hypnosis, Reiki and emotional freedom techniques (tapping), meditation, and massage. Explore the American Holistic Nurses Association website www.ahna.org and the National Center for Complementary and Alternative Medicine http://nccam.nih.gov/health/whatiscam.

• Diversify, diversify, diversify. While following a patient to cardiac rehab, did you get excited about the possibilities of working there? If so, explore potential opportunities.

• Be flexible. Cast a wide net when considering different opportunities. The options are endless. Consider case management, telephone triage, pharmaceutical sales, research, medical coding, medical transcription, legal nurse consulting, parish nursing, teaching, informatics, quality assurance, writing for healthcare-related publications, and school or camp nursing.

• Take care of your finances. Consider disability insurance and invest wisely (payroll deductions, IRAs). Save for that rainy day. Invest in mortgage and credit unemployment insurance, and set money aside in liquid assets—preferably at least six months' worth of income. This way, you have the cash to survive an interruption in income, and the unemployment insurance will ensure that your home and credit cards are protected during this time. The results of the nurse retirement study conducted by Fidelity Investments (2013) show that most nurses are not confident they will have enough savings to retire.

• Read and listen. Find out about new career opportunities in nursing. Attend Donna Cardillo's Career Alternatives for Nurses™ seminar or purchase a DVD, audiocassette, or videotape of the presentation. After her presentation, you'll feel good and positive about yourself and your profession and be armed with information, resources, and motivation to move forward in your career.

• Consider a career coach. A life or career coach may help you achieve your goals. For instance, Carmen Kosicek has a wealth of experience helping nurses find positions outside of the hospital. http://carmenkosicek.com/.

• Write. Following a back injury, Trenee' Carlson Zweigle (2004), wrote *Psych Ward*, a book about her experiences working in mental health settings and later she wrote *Never Give Up: Hope and Encouragement for Women* (2013). Patricia Holloran (2005) wrote *Walking Like a Duck* based on her personal journey from addiction to recovery. Following a work-related spinal injury, Anne Hudson and William Charney (2003) wrote *Back Injury Among Healthcare Workers*. An article by Carolyn McKinzie (2012), appears in the Amputee Coalition's magazine *In Motion*. Cleo Graham (2005) wrote a book called *From Mess to Message Understanding the Hidden Meanings of Pain and Suffering*. Christine Molloy (2013) wrote *Tales from the Dry Side: The Personal Stories Behind the Autoimmune Illness Sjögren's Syndrome*. Karen Ingalls (2012) wrote a book about her journey with ovarian cancer. It is called *Outshine: An Ovarian Cancer Memoir*. Susan Fleming (2014) wrote a book about her grandmother called *Alice Ada Wood Ellis: Seattle Pioneer Midwife, Nurse, & Mother to All*. Based on her experiences as a nurse with dystonia, Beka Serdans wrote a book called *I'm Moving On…Are U?* (2001). She also wrote

I'm Moving, Too: A Poetic Journey with Dystonia (2000).

- Keep a journal. Journal writing is helpful to many people. Through guided questions, Ritter (2006) developed a workbook that helps to develop a self-care plan for people suffering from the loss of physical capacity. The exercises help people see how they still have strengths and abilities and can move beyond being disabled. It encourages readers not to wallow on what has been lost.

- Become your own publicist. Stories about nurses with disabilities are important. Contact your local newspaper, radio, or television station. Ask them to consider doing an interview with you. Write a letter to the editor of your local newspaper. Positive, uplifting stories about successful accommodations and working with a disability will help others and bring positive attention to your place of employment. If you are not working and want to work, share your story.

- Blog. Write a blog about your experiences as a nurse or nursing student with a disability. Exceptional Nurse has a blog that can be found at http://exceptionalnurse.blogspot.com/. Carolyn McKinzie, LPN, who has an amputation (see Chapter 13) writes a blog for the Abled Amputees of America www.abledamputees.org/#!heart-of-inspiration/csv7

- Start a nonprofit organization. Rebecca Serdans, RN is challenged by dystonia. She created the nonprofit organization Care4Dystonia that focuses on patient care and building awareness. www.care4dystonia.org.

- Mentor others. Pay it forward. If you started your nursing career with a disability, write and speak about your experiences. Tell others how you accomplished your goal. Mentor other nurses and nursing students with disabilities.

- Get involved in a disability organization. There may be a future career path within a disability related organization. Detra Bannister (who commented in this book) was a school nurse. Her vision loss led to a position as a CareerConnect specialist with the American Foundation for the Blind. Detra assists nurses and others with vision loss to find or maintain employment (Maheady, 2011)

• Use social media to connect with other nurses—with and without disabilities. Sign up for newsletters, join discussion groups, and participate in webinars or webcasts.

• Adjunct. Opportunities to develop or teach courses taught via the Internet are endless. Consider teaching a clinical course. Marianne Haugh, RN, was born with spina bifida. She uses a wheelchair and is a nursing clinical instructor for Harper College and the University of St. Francis (Pecci, 2013).

• Research. Conduct research about the experiences of nurses with disabilities. Consider this topic for a master's or doctoral dissertation. Grants are available to support this type of inquiry.

• Develop a life outside of nursing. Spend time with family and friends. Participate in sporting activities. Join a Bunko group, book club, or knitting group. Attend plays and cultural events. Travel. Get a life beyond the walls of your unit.

• Be prepared to relocate to another area. Perhaps a warmer climate, slower pace, or a city with good public transportation would be a good move. Think about places you would and would not want to live.

• Stay abreast of national and international disability online networks. Many websites for people who have disabilities post advertisements for employment. Through these networks, there may be people already connected to the local job market in your career field who could provide you with valuable information about the market and possible employment opportunities.

• Conduct a periodic job search and develop self-promotion strategies. Keep your resume or portfolio current. Attend career fairs in your area. Create a professional online network (LinkedIn, Facebook or other social media websites). Be prepared and ready to interview on short notice.

• Start a business. Latrell Castanon, RN, started a business called Servant Nurse Staffing in Lubbock, Texas. Thelma Stich started a business offering student nurse tutoring www.studentnursetutor.com. Visit the National Nurses in Business www.nnba.net to formulate ideas or take a course. Or, visit The Nurse Entrepreneur Website www.nursefriendly.com/nursing/business.htm to learn about entrepreneurial opportunities.

• Keep your spiritual side vibrant. Get or stay involved with a religious or spiritual group. If organized religion is part of your life, consider becoming a parish nurse in the denomination of your choice, be it at a church, synagogue, temple, or mosque. Enjoy doing yoga? Consider becoming a certified yoga nurse by taking a course with Annette Tersigni, RN. http://yoganurse.com/.

• Surround yourself with positive people. Nurture positive interpersonal relationships in your work setting. Be as nonconfrontational as possible. Remember the dictum: You can catch more flies with honey than you can with vinegar. Extend small kindnesses to others. Should someone be rude, smile back, and show them a better way. This attitude helps make everyone's experience better. Positive attitudes make all the difference in most of life's activities.

Building Resilience

Don't give up your nursing license

Stay healthy: mentally and physically

Network

Volunteer

Stay current with technology

Learn new skills

Continue your education

Diversify, diversify, diversify

Have a Plan "B"

Donna Carol Maheady, ARNP, EdD, the mother of an adult daughter with autism and related disabilities, is a board certified Pediatric Nurse Practitioner and an Associate Graduate Faculty member in the Christine E. Lynn College of Nursing at Florida Atlantic University. Dr. Maheady has conducted research on the experiences of nursing students with disabilities, published numerous articles and is the author of Nursing Students with Disabilities Change the Course *(winner of the American Journal of Nursing 2004 Book of the Year Award)* and Leave No Nurse Behind: Nurses working with disAbilities. *She is the founder of the nonprofit resource network www.ExceptionalNurse.com and can be reached at ExceptionalNurse@aol.com.*

References

Adleman, C. S. (2005). Writing your way to health and healing: An interactive workshop. Retrieved on December 16, 2013 at http://exceptionalnurse.com/pdf/ONLINEWORKSHOPFORNURSES.pdf.

Adleman, C. S. (2005). Recovering from stroke: A journey toward health. Retrieved on December 16, 2013 at http://www.exceptionalnurse.com/FLTarticlewithsidebars.pdf.

Cardillo, D. Career alternatives for nurses®

http://donnacardillo.com/shop/career-alternatives-for-nurses/

Charney, W. & Hudson, A. (2003). *Back injury among healthcare workers*. Boca Raton, FL: CRC Press.

Fidelity Investments (2013). *Fidelity® study shows increase in nurses' retirement savings, yet many not confident they will have enough to retire.* Retrieved on December 20, 2013 at http://www.fidelity.com/inside-fidelity/individual-investing/fidelity-study-shows-increase

Fleming, S. (2014). *Alice Ada Wood Ellis: Seattle pioneer midwife, nurse, & mother to all.* Createspace.com.

Graham, C. (2005). *From mess to message: Understanding the hidden meanings of pain and suffering.* Amazon Digital Services.

Holloran, P. (2005). *Walking like a duck: The true story of a nurse walking from addiction to recovery.* Lincoln, NE: iUniverse.

Ingalls, K. (2012). *Outshine: An ovarian cancer memoir.* Edina, Minnesota: Beaver's Pond Press.

Lynch, J. P. (2013). Red Cross condolence program volunteers help families need. Nurse.com. Retrieved on December 18, 2013 at http://news.nurse.com/article/20130506/NY02/105060039?sf12678185=1#.UrCJuXKA3q5.

Maheady, D. (2011). *Shedding light on nurses with vision loss.* Nursetogether.com. Retrieved on December 18, 2013 at www.nursetogether.com/shedding-light-on-nurses-with-vision-loss

McKinzie, C. (2012). Recovery and Reunion: A mother and daughter's reflections on the long journey back. In Motion, 22 (1) 30-31. Retrieved on September 16 from www.amputee-coalition.org/inmotion_online/inmotion-22-01-web/pubData/source/jan-feb_2012fb.pdf.

Molloy, C. (2013). *Tales from the dry side: The personal stories behind the autoimmune illness Sjögren's Syndrome.* Outskirts Press.

Pecci, A. (2013). Give nurses in wheelchairs a chance. *Health Leaders Media.* Retrieved on December 17, 2013 at www.healthleadersmedia.com/page-1/NRS-299106/Give-Nurses-in-Wheelchairs-a-Chance

Ritter, R. (2006). *Coping with physical loss and disability.* Ann Arbor, MI: Loving Healing Press.

Serdans, B. (2001). *I'm moving on…are U?* Philadelphia, PA: Xlibris Corporation.

Serdans, B. (2000). *I'm moving two.* Philadelphia, PA: Xlibris Corporation.

Zweigle, T.C. (2005). *Psych ward.* Frederick, MD: Publish America.

Zweigle, T. C. (2013). *Never give up: Hope and encouragement for women.* CreateSpace.com.

CONCLUSION

By Donna Carol Maheady, ARNP, EdD

All nurses need to consider the possibility of illness or disability in their long-term career planning. No one knows when an injury, illness, natural disaster, or a mental or physical condition will leave him or her with a disability. But ongoing continuing education, the pursuit of advanced degrees, current certifications, flexibility, thinking outside of the box, and a positive attitude will increase employability options whether or not you ever become disabled.

If disability is or becomes part of your life, know you are not alone. Get connected with others. And if you need to use a cane, decorate it! Be honest with yourself and make a plan. Paint your paradise. Take charge of your future. What would you like to do? Make a list of your strengths, interests, experience, education, needs, and limitations. Compare your list with various nursing job descriptions. Where do you fit best?

Whether you are a student pursuing a nursing degree, a nurse struggling with a disability, or a hospital administrator called on to accommodate a nurse, creativity is the key to success. There is always another way to accomplish any given task: Find it.

Nurses are intelligent, caring, and creative problem solvers. Daily, they assist patients in navigating the healthcare system and adjusting to disability and illness. As evidenced through the stories shared, nurses with disabilities have much to offer patient care. They can be an asset to institutions where they are employed because they can identify with a patient's thoughts, feelings, and concerns. They have "been there" and "done that" on both sides of nursing care. They understand what patients want in a nurse. They have also had to work to combat discrimination and physical limitations and still have the guts and know-how that nursing calls for.

Nurses with disabilities are entitled to request and receive reasonable accommodation to enable them to perform the essential functions of a job. Furthermore, they have the right to equal enjoyment of the benefits and privileges of employment enjoyed by others. Unfortunately, nurses with disabilities still encounter a great deal of stigma. But by knowing the law, nurses with disabilities can take action to ensure that they are afforded opportunities equal to other nurses.

If you need accommodations to be successful in your job, the key is to remember is that employers are only obliged to grant accommodations if you ask and they need to be reasonable requests. Be prepared to justify your request and explain why it's in the employer's best interest to grant it. Often accommodations can be simple and low in cost. If the accommodation request is costly, develop and share a cost/benefit summary. Compare the cost of recruitment and hiring a new nurse or travel nurse with the cost included in your request.

Some accommodations can be provided informally and offered simply as helpful gestures from colleagues. In supportive environments, all a nurse may need is for a colleague to extend a helping hand. When helpful gestures are offered to you, try to return the gesture whenever possible. By making sure your disability is not associated with a difficult working situation for others, you can more readily gain acceptance.

While it's vital—both for your safety and that of your patients—to know your limitations, it's also important to realize that you may have to work harder than colleagues without disabilities to overcome stereotypes and gain their respect. Be prepared to have to prove yourself often over and over. Don't be afraid to ask for help when you need it, but be willing to lend a hand in return whenever it's needed of you. Give as much as you take.

Flexibility Matters

Don't give up on a dream because you have a disability. Find another way to achieve it. Sometimes that means persevering in a current job to prove to your coworkers and hospital administrators that it can be done. Other times, it may mean being more flexible by considering different areas of nursing or finding new ways to use your knowledge outside of direct patient care.

Sometimes, a disability can open new doors for you—but only if you are willing to see those possibilities. You may be blinded to them if you only dwell on what you have lost as a result of your condition. Seek out other nurses in similar situations. Don't push away. As Sheryl Sandberg (2013), CEO of Facebook and bestselling author states "Lean In."

Be Your Own Advocate

Make sure your employer knows how your disability makes you an especially valuable member of the team. Be your own champion. Keep your eyes open to every possibility along the way. Writing, public speaking, and bringing positive media attention to your place of employment can be helpful. As a nurse, you are used to being an advocate for your patients. Do the same for yourself. Sharing your story will help you as the teller and others as listeners to gain insight into being resilient and the strength needed to cope with a challenging life event.

Don't be afraid to use assertiveness to nudge things forward with human resources, administrators, university or college disability service staffers or state vocational rehabilitation counselors. By having the patience and willingness to educate others about how much a person with a disability can accomplish, you can pave the way for yourself and other nurses with disabilities as well.

Nursing administrators need to have greater awareness of the struggles of some of their colleagues to continue practicing. Many nurses are underemployed and long to return to work. Why not give one an interview? And, ask how he or she could do the job? Turn to other administrators who have hired a similarly situated nurse. Ask about accommodations. What worked and what could have worked better? Keep an open mind.

Administrators and human resource staffers should facilitate accommodations for more nurses with disabilities. Employment advertisements should state: "Nurses with disabilities encouraged to apply." Applicants need to be considered individually, based on their abilities, not their limitations. And accommodation plans should be developed that assess essential functions, particularly lifting and CPR in a new light. Some questions to ask include: Is performance of CPR essential to the nursing position being considered? Or, is safe patient handling and mobility equipment available?

Nurses need to reach out to colleagues with disabilities and encourage them to stay or invite them to come back to work. Parents of children with disabilities need to encourage their children to follow their dreams which may include a career in nursing. Pediatric nurses caring for children with chronic illness and disabilities need to recognize that a future nurse may be in their hands.

State nursing boards should examine or re-examine rules and regulations regarding licensure of nurses with disabilities. The mental health needs of nurses who work through disasters and other traumatic events need to be acknowledged more. And, employee assistance programs need to be improved in order to live up to their promises.

Organizations that employ nurses with disabilities and welcome nursing students with disabilities to clinical experiences send powerful, supportive messages to their patients and communities. There's hope after illness or disability. I can have a career; I can have a life after this.

State vocational rehabilitation programs need to collaborate more with nurse leaders and nursing education programs and recognize the vast opportunities within the nursing profession beyond the bedside. Often educational support for a nurse to obtain an advanced degree can mean the difference between a life on disability assistance and a productive life as a nurse.

Additionally, nursing programs need to create more diverse, accommodating academic programs. Nurses and educators need to reach out to students with disabilities, cultivate their passion, harvest the potential, and welcome them. A collaborative spirit needs to be developed and nurtured between nursing faculty members and college or university disability services staffers.

Colleges and universities also need to hire more nurses with disabilities to teach in their nursing programs. Nursing faculty with disabilities have much to contribute to student learning in face-to-face and online classes and clinical settings. They also serve as role models for nursing students with disabilities.

Nurses need to look at the seat next to them at the nurse's station, office or community setting… move over, and make room for a nurse with a disability to find a seat. There is more than enough room for nurses with disabilities within the profession—not just because of the Americans with Disabilities Act, the nursing shortage, litigation, or a workers' compensation claim—but simply because it's the right thing to do.

Nurses with disabilities don't have to live down to the disability stereotype. They should hold their heads high, fully prepared with the knowledge that discrimination exists, but also aware that it doesn't have to close the door. Nursing with a disability can be a challenge, but it is not impossible. The nurses who have shared their stories are living proof. A sense of humor, perseverance, a positive attitude, and—resilience—helped these nurses continue to practice and thrive. Working helps nurses with disabilities maintain independence, health, and self-esteem. At the end of the day, they have worked—and benefitted their patients and themselves.

So, what are you waiting for? Disability doesn't always mean the end. Often it is the beginning. If it happens to you, don't be defined by the disability; be defined by how you handle it.

Reference

Sandberg, S. (2013). *Lean in: Women, work and the will to lead.* New York: Knopf.

CLOSING AFFIRMATIONS

By Connie Stallone Adleman, RN

I'd like to offer each nurse who has a disability, the following affirmations:

I use my limitations as an opportunity to grow.

I give thanks that any limitation that I experience is a gift teaching me about myself.

I always focus on and count my possibilities for success.

I have unlimited potential.

I love myself exactly as I am.

APPENDIX A

Sample Accommodation Request Letter

The following is an example of what can be included in an accommodation request letter. It is not intended to be legal advice:

Date of Letter
Your name
Your address
Employer's name
Employer's address

Dear (e.g., Supervisor, Manager, Human Resources, Personnel):

Content to consider in body of letter:
Identify yourself as a person with a disability.
State that you are requesting accommodations under the ADA (or the Rehabilitation Act of 1973 if you are a federal employee).
Identify your specific problematic job tasks.
Identify your accommodation ideas.
Request your employer's accommodation ideas.
Refer to attached medical documentation if appropriate.*
Ask that your employer respond to your request in a reasonable amount of time.

Sincerely,
Your signature

Your printed name
Cc: To appropriate individuals

You may want to attach medical information to your letter to help establish that you are a person with a disability and to document the need for accommodation.

* Source: Department of Labor, Office of Disability Employment Policy, Job Accommodation Network
http://askjan.org/media/downloads/accommodationrequestletter.pdf

APPENDIX B

Disclosing Your Psychiatric Disability to an Employer

Only you can decide whether and how much to tell your employer about your psychiatric disability. On the positive side, telling your employer about your diagnosis is the only way to protect your legal right to any accommodations you might need to get or keep a job. However, revealing your disability also leaves you open to discrimination, which may limit your opportunities for employment and advancement. It's a complex decision and one you shouldn't make until you've thought it through. Here's what you might want to think about:

Preparing to Disclose

Assess your job search skills to determine whether you need help from your therapist or mental health agency to:

- Initiate contact or arrange an interview with the employer.

- Interview.

- Describe your disability.

- Negotiate the terms of employment.

- Negotiate accommodations.

1. Identify any potential accommodations you might need during the hiring process or on your first day of work.

2. Explore your feelings about having a mental illness and about sharing that information with others. Remember, no one can force you to disclose if you don't want to.

3. Research potential employers' attitudes toward mental illness and screen out unsupportive employers. Consider:

- Have they hired someone with a psychiatric disability before?

- Do they personally know someone with a mental illness?

- What positive or negative experiences have they had in employing someone with a mental illness?

- Do they show signs—in newsletters, posted notices, employee education programs about mental illness, etc. —of encouraging a diverse workforce?

- Do they have a corporate culture that favors flextime, mentoring, telecommuting, flexible benefit plans, and other programs that help employees work efficiently and well?

- Does the job have certain requirements (e.g., childcare or high security) that would put you at a disadvantage if you disclosed your diagnosis?

4. Weigh the benefits and risks of disclosure:

- Do you need to involve an outside agency to get or keep the job?

- Do you need accommodation or other employer support?

- When will you need this accommodation?

- Do other people in the company need similar accommodation?

- How stressful will it be for you to hide your disability?

5. If you decide not to disclose, find other ways to get the support you need:

- Seek out behind-the-scenes support from friends, therapists, etc.

- Research potential employers who provide this support to all employees.

6. If you decide to disclose, plan in advance how you'll handle it:

- Who will say it (you, your therapist, your job coach, etc.)?

- What to say (see below)?

- When to say it?

Under the ADA, a person with a disability can choose to disclose at any time and is not required to disclose at all unless he wants to request an accommodation or wants other protection under the law. Someone with a disability can disclose at any of these times:

- Before the hiring interview.

- During the interview.

- After the interview, but before any job offer.

- After a job offer, but before starting a job.

- Anytime after beginning a job.

We recommend disclosing sometime before serious problems arise on the job. It is unlikely that you would be protected under the ADA if you disclosed right before you were about to get fired. Employers are most likely to be responsive to a disclosure if they think it is done in good faith and not as a last-ditch effort to keep your job. Who you should tell:

- Your supervisor or manager, if he must provide or approve an accommodation.

- The EEO/affirmative action officer or human resources staff, if no immediate accommodation is needed but you would like the protection of the ADA.

- The person interviewing you or human resources staff, if you might need accommodation during the hiring process.

- The employee assistance program staff, if you are already on the job, experiencing difficulties, and need help deciding how, how much, and to whom to disclose.

When You Disclose

1. Decide how specific you will be in describing your psychiatric disability:

    - In general terms: a disability, a medical condition, or an illness.

    - In vague but more specific terms: a biochemical imbalance, a neurological problem, a brain disorder, or difficulty with stress.

    - More specifically referring to mental illness: a mental illness, psychiatric disorder, or mental disability.

    - Your exact diagnosis: schizophrenia, bipolar disorder, major depression, or anxiety disorder.

2. Describe the skills you have that make you able to perform the main duties of the job.

    - Qualifications

    - Technical skills

    - General work skills

3. Describe any functional limitations or behaviors caused by your disability that interfere with your performance (See Steps to Define Functional Limitations).

4. Identify the accommodations you need to overcome those functional limitations or behaviors (See Steps to Identify Reasonable Accommodations).

5. Optional: You may choose to describe the behaviors or symptoms the employer might observe and tell the employer what steps to take as a result.

6. Point the employer to resources for further information:

    - Employment specialist, supported employment provider, rehabilitation counselor or job coach

    - Doctor or psychiatrist

- Therapist, counselor or social worker

- Job Accommodation Network

- ADA Disability and Business Technical Assistance Centers

- Others listed in the Resources Section.

7. You may find it helpful to prepare a script to read from. For example:

- "I have (preferred term for psychiatric disability) that I am recovering from. Currently, I can/have (the skills required) to do (the main duties) of the job, but sometimes (functional limitations) interfere with my ability to (duties you may have trouble performing). It helps if I have (name the specific accommodations you need). I work best when (other accommodations)."

8. You could also add the following information:

- "Sometimes you might see (symptoms or behaviors associated with symptoms). When you see that, you can (name the action steps for the employer). Here is the number of my (employment specialist, doctor, therapist, previous employer, JAN, etc.) for any information that you might need about my ability to handle the job."

© 1997, 1998 Center for Psychiatric Rehabilitation, Boston University.

http://cpr.bu.edu/resources/reasonable-accommodations/jobschool/disclosing-your-disability-to-an-employer

APPENDIX C

Guide to Requesting State Vocational Rehabilitation Services
By Cheryl Machemer, MSN, RN, CCRN-CSC

Note: The state vocational rehabilitation services office will determine what services, if any, will be awarded to the nursing student/professional nurse. This is meant to be a guide to organize a request related to hearing loss. It could be adapted for any disability.

Request for support from the (State)_____Vocational Rehabilitation Services Office

Name: _____

Date:_____

Contact Information: Email: _____ Phone: _____

Mailing Address: _____

_____

Nursing Student ___Professional Nurse___

Client/Case Number: _____

Describe your personal background/ situation. Why are you requesting services from Vocational Rehabilitation?

Education: Nursing Assistant_____ Licensed Practical Nurse_____
Associate Degree_____
Bachelor's Degree in Nursing_____ Master's Degree in Nursing_____
Additional certifications _____

Disability
Type of Hearing Loss:
___ Hearing Loss Since Birth ___ Late Deafened ___Hard-of-Hearing
___Profoundly Deaf
___ Low Pitched Loss   ___ High Pitched loss

____ Hearing Loss Occurred Before Language Development ____ Hearing Loss Occurred After   Language Development

Assistive Devices used:

Hearing Aid____ Behind the Ear ____ In the Ear ____In the Canal___Completely in Canal___
Cochlear Implant ___Surgical Implant___

Stethoscope currently used:

____ Traditional ___Digital ___Bluetooth Capable ___Visual Stethoscope ___Stethoscope with Headphones

Accommodations needed:

____ Lip reading ___ CART (Communication Access Real Time) ___FM System
____ American Sign Language (ASL) ___Interpretive Services ___Note Taker
____ Front row seating ___TYY (Texting Telephone) ____ Recorded Lectures
____ Clear Surgical Masks ___ iPad for Communication ____ Taped Report

Related issues:

____ Mobility (loss of balance, coordination, dizziness)
____ Background noise affects hearing
____ Vision loss
____ Difficulty interacting with peers
____ Speech difficulty
____ Delayed comprehension when spoken to
____ Difficulty hearing classmates/teacher in the classroom
____ Difficulty hearing patient call bells/ monitor alarms
____ Difficulty hearing others speaking on the nursing unit/ operating room

___ Difficulty hearing on the telephone
___ Fatigue
___ Denial of hearing loss
___ Frequently asking others to repeat themselves
___ Unfamiliar with how to care for hearing aid

Current Employment

Hospital, clinic, doctor's office_____ Specialty
area_____.
Do you plan to stay on this unit? In this specialty area? Do you intend to
continue your education?

Student

Indicate the school you are currently attending or have applied to, date
accepted, and expected date of graduation.

Student or Nurse

State your long-term career goals. Include any volunteer experience, places
of employment and length time in each position, and any other information
that may be helpful for the vocational rehabilitation counselor. *Help the
counselor help you.

Goal: To complete the Certified Nursing Assistant ___LPN/ LVN;
___Diploma; ___ADN; ___BSN; ___ MSN; ___DNP; ___ PhD program.
Upon completion of this program, what do you plan to do?
Where do you plan to work? (maternal child health, emergency nursing,
operating room, education, case management, legal nurse consulting?)

*** Include statistics, articles, books, and resources to strengthen your
application. Attach scholarly journal articles documenting examples of
nurses practicing with hearing loss or articles about nurses with hearing loss
practicing in different roles.

Cheryl Machemer, MSN, RN, CCRN-CSC teaches nursing at the Reading Hospital School of Health Sciences, Nursing Program, The Reading Hospital and Medical Center, Reading, PA. She was diagnosed with moderate to severe bilateral sensorineural hearing loss at the age of 40 and wears bilateral behind-the-ear hearing aids. Cheryl has a master's of science degree in nursing with a concentration in nursing education from Kutztown University. Her thesis examined the lived experience of the hearing-impaired nursing student. She is a board member and the nurse professional leader for the Association of Medical Professionals with Hearing Losses (www.amphl.org) and member of www.ExceptionalNurse.com. Cheryl can be reached at cherylmachemer@gmail.com.

RESOURCES

Organizations

ExceptionalNurse.com

A nonprofit resource network for nursing students and nurses with disabilities. www.ExceptionalNurse.com.

Exceptional Nurse Group on Facebook
https://www.facebook.com/groups/ExceptionalNurse/

Exceptional Nurse Blog http://exceptionalnurse.blogspot.com/

Exceptional Nurse on LinkedIn http://www.linkedin.com/

Exceptional Nurse on Twitter www.Twitter.com/ExceptNurse

Association of Medical Professionals with Hearing Loss

www.AMPHL.org A network for individuals with hearing losses working in the health care field.

UK Health Professionals with Hearing Loss

http://hphl.org.uk/ Health professionals who are d/Deaf share information and support in the United Kingdom.

Association of Nurses in Aids Care

Provides information for HIV+ nurses and students. http://www.nursesinaidscare.org/files/public/Nursing_Student_F AQ_2010.pdf

Reasonable Accommodations

Office of the Americans with Disabilities Act

www.usdoj.gov/crt/ada/adahom1.htm

Southern Regional Education Board

The Southern Regional Education Board Council on Collegiate Education for Nursing Education published— The Americans with Disabilities Act: Implications for Nursing Education —to help nurse educators comply with the 1990 Americans with Disabilities Act (ADA).
http://www.sreb.org/page/1390/the_americans_with_disabilities_act.html

The U.S. Equal Employment Opportunity Commission

www.eeoc.gov/policy/guidance.html

The EEOC provides information about reasonable accommodations and other aspects of the ADA.

Telework as a Reasonable Accommodation

www.eeoc.gov./facts/telework.html

The Equal Employment Opportunity Commission offers a fact sheet that explains the ways that employers can allow an individual to work at home as a reasonable accommodation.

Job Accommodation Network

http://askjan.org/links/about.htm

The Job Accommodation Network (JAN) counselors perform individualized searches for workplace accommodations.

JAN published the *Occupation and Industry Series: Accommodating Nurses with Disabilities.* http://askjan.org/media/nurses.html

Service Animals

http://www.ada.gov/service_animals_2010.htm

The U.S. Department of Justice provides guidance on service animals.

Family Medical Leave

http://www.dol.gov/dol/topic/benefits-leave/fmla.htm

The U.S. Department of Labor provides general information about family medical leave.

Mental Health

Center for Psychiatric Rehabilitation

http://www.bu.edu/cpr/reasaccom/

Offers assistance to employers and educators related to reasonable accommodation for people with psychiatric disabilities.

Hearing Loss

PEPNet.org

www.PepNet.org

The Postsecondary Education Programs Network is the national collaboration of the four Regional Postsecondary Education Centers for Individuals who are Deaf and Hard of Hearing.

Self Help for Hard of Hearing People, Inc.

www.shhh.org/

Provides information about listening devices, education, support and advocacy.

Phonic Ear

www.phonicear.com

This company provides a variety of listening devices for people with hearing loss.

Learning Disabilities

National Library Service for the Blind and Physically Handicapped

www.loc.gov/nls

The service provides free recorded and Braille reading materials to persons with visual or physical impairments that prevent the reading of standard print material.

Learning Ally

https://www.learningally.org/

Learning Ally is a provider of audiobooks to students with learning disabilities.

Reading Pen

This device provides people with reading difficulties, learning disabilities or dyslexia with immediate word support.
http://www.wizcomtech.com/Wizcom/products/products.asp?fid=78

Financial Assistance

Social Security Administration

www.ssa.gov

The Social Security Administration provides benefits to persons with a physical or mental disability that prevents them from working.

Nurseshouse.org

Web site: www.Nurseshouse.org

Offers temporary financial assistance to nurses who are ill, convalescing or disabled.

Vocational Rehabilitation (VR)

Vocational Rehabilitation is a nationwide federal-state program for assisting eligible people with disabilities to become employed. VR provides counseling, education, training, and other support services. http://www.vba.va.gov/bln/vre

Department of Veterans Affairs

http://www.vba.va.gov/bln/vre/

The Department of Veterans Affairs provides counseling and services to service-connected disabled veterans.

Stethoscopes and Blood Pressure Monitors

Stethoscopes.com

Web site: www.stethoscopes.com

This web site offers a variety of stethoscopes for people with hearing loss.

Welch Allyn

Web site: www.welchallyn.com

This company distributes a variety of special stethoscopes and medical equipment.

Allheart.com

Web site: www.allheart.com

This company provides amplified stethoscopes for people with hearing loss.

Ultrascopes.com

www.ultrascopes.com

The pressure sensitive 'Ultrascope" is available for people with hearing loss.

Cardionics Inc.

www.cardionics.com

This company manufactures the "E" Scope and Pocket Monitor for people with hearing loss.

The pocket monitor provides a visual display of heart and lung sounds on a personal digital assistant (PDA).

ThinkLabs One

An electromagnetic diaphragm is key to the audio quality of every ThinkLabs digital stethoscope.

http://www.thinklabs.com/

Stethoscope Holster

The holster holds a stethoscope in a variety of configurations taking weight off the neck area.

http://www.nurseborn.com

One-Hand Blood Pressure Monitors

One-hand aneroid blood pressure monitors are available from many companies. The pump and dial are attached to the same handle and can be manipulated with one hand.

Vision Loss

Sight Connection

www.sightconnection.com

This company provides talking blood pressure monitors, talking thermometers, and talking scales.

Standing Wheelchairs

Levo

http://levousa.com/

This company has been engaged in the development, production and distribution of stand-up wheelchairs.

See-Through Surgical Masks

The Association of Medical Professional with Hearing Loss

www.AMPHL.org. provides information about the progress of production and availability of see-through surgical masks.

Computers and related equipment

IBM Accessibility Center

www.ibm.com/able/

Provides information on how IBM products can assist people disabilities use personal computers.

Apple Computers

http://www.apple.com/support/accessibility/

Provides a wide range of hardware and software to assist people with special needs.

Microsoft

www.microsoft.com/enable/default.aspx

A wide range of accessibility technology is available for people with disabilities.

Mouse adapter

Enables people who suffer from hand tremors to eliminate excessive cursor movement. It is available from Montrose Secam Limited.
http://www.montrosesecam.com/

Video Clips

Danielle's story

Born missing a limb from her elbow, Danielle found ways to succeed in nursing school, graduate and land a job as a pediatric nurse.

http://www.youtube.com/watch?v=9h8y9WICHu4

Dyslexic nurse refuses to let reading problems stand in her way

http://www.youtube.com/watch?v=p1IiajxUIf0

Nursing with the hand you are given

Susan Fleming, RN, PhD, born missing her left hand demonstrates nursing skills

http://www.youtube.com/watch?v=d3AfRRNxLWg

The Disabled Nurse: Focus on Abilities

http://vimeo.com/20809344

Nursing math: Do not let the math stop you from becoming a nurse

http://www.youtube.com/watch?v=0QaN1BvI3Vk&feature=youtu.be

A nurse with a learning disability shares her remarkable journey

http://icould.com/videos/marie-e/

CPSIA information can be obtained
at www.ICGtesting.com
Printed in the USA
LVOW13s2040130617

537969LV00019B/203/P